Teaching Qualitative Research in Public Health

AF386008

TEACHING PUBLIC HEALTH

Teaching Public Health offers instructors state-of-the-science tools and resources to support integration of new topics and pedagogical strategies that can promote active, engaged, and innovative learning in academic public health.

SERIES EDITORS
LISA SULLIVAN, *Boston University School of Public Health*
SANDRO GALEA, *Boston University School of Public Health*

Teaching Public Health Writing
Jennifer Beard

Teaching Qualitative Research in Public Health
Katherine Clegg Smith, Jill Owczarzak, Caitlin Kennedy, and Shannon Frattaroli

Teaching Qualitative Research in Public Health

Katherine Clegg Smith
Jill Owczarzak
Caitlin Kennedy
Shannon Frattaroli

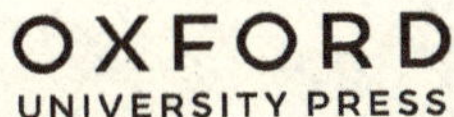

OXFORD
UNIVERSITY PRESS

OXFORD
UNIVERSITY PRESS

Oxford University Press is a department of the University of Oxford.
It furthers the University's objective of excellence in research, scholarship,
and education by publishing worldwide. Oxford is a registered trade mark of
Oxford University Press in the UK and in certain other countries.

Published in the United States of America by Oxford University Press
198 Madison Avenue, New York, NY 10016, United States of America.

© Oxford University Press 2026

All rights reserved. No part of this publication may be reproduced, stored in a retrieval system,
transmitted, used for text and data mining, or used for training artificial intelligence, in any form or
by any means, without the prior permission in writing of Oxford University Press, or as expressly
permitted by law, by license, or under terms agreed with the appropriate reprographics rights
organization. Inquiries concerning reproduction outside the scope of the above should be sent
to the Rights Department, Oxford University Press, at the address above.

You must not circulate this work in any other form
and you must impose this same condition on any acquirer.

CIP data is on file at the Library of Congress.

This material is not intended to be, and should not be considered, a substitute for medical or other
professional advice. Treatment for the conditions described in this material is highly dependent on
the individual circumstances. And, while this material is designed to offer accurate information with
respect to the subject matter covered and to be current as of the time it was written, research and
knowledge about medical and health issues are constantly evolving and dose schedules for medications
are being revised continually, with new side effects recognized and accounted for regularly. Readers
must therefore always check the product information and clinical procedures with the most up-to-date
published product information and data sheets provided by the manufacturers and the most recent
codes of conduct and safety regulations. The publisher and the authors make no representations or
warranties to readers, express or implied, as to the accuracy or completeness of this material. Without
limiting the foregoing, the publisher and the authors make no representations or warranties as to the
accuracy or efficacy of the drug dosages mentioned in the material. The authors and the publisher do
not accept, and expressly disclaim, any responsibility for any liability, loss, or risk that may be claimed or
incurred as a consequence of the use and/ or application of any of the contents of this material.

ISBN 9780197662441

DOI: 10.1093/9780197662472.001.0001

Printed by Marquis Book Printing, Canada

The manufacturer's authorized representative in the EU for product safety is
Oxford University Press España S.A. of Parque Empresarial San Fernando de Henares,
Avenida de Castilla, 2 – 28830 Madrid (www.oup.es/en or product.safety@oup.com).
OUP España S.A. also acts as importer into Spain of products made by the manufacturer.

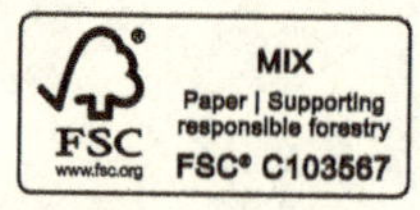

Contents

List of Figures

List of Tables

List of Boxes

Series Foreword

Academic public health has been growing substantially over the past two decades. There are increasingly more accredited schools and programs of public health, and more stand-alone baccalaureate programs. Teaching in academic public health similarly continues to grow at both the undergraduate and graduate levels, with more faculty engaged in public health education, research, and practice.

Coincident with this growth in interest in the field, established graduate schools and programs of public health are redesigning curricula to meet the changing needs of incoming students and to ensure that graduates have the knowledge, skills, and attributes to meet the needs of a changing workforce. A cornerstone of these revised curricula, in line with evolving accreditation standards set by the Council on Education for Public Health, is integrating knowledge across disciplines to teach students that the foundations of public health do not exist in disciplinary silos but rather need to be addressed at the interstices of disciplines.

However, teaching public health across disciplines can present challenges for instructors, many of whom are new and bring different areas of expertise to public health. It often requires using different books with insights from across disciplines and finding ways to integrate material that is not being integrated in any one book. In addition, the material across integrative areas of study evolves quickly, making it difficult, if not impossible, for one definitive textbook to cover all that needs to be covered across several integrative courses.

Recognizing both the potential in burgeoning public health training and the challenges and opportunities presented by more integrative learning, we propose *Teaching Public Health: An Integrated*

Approach, a series of primers for faculty teaching public health or for professionals to learn essential concepts.

The series will provide instructors with tools and techniques to meet educational trends including online and other more flexible teaching and learning modalities, design of stackable credentials building to degrees, on-demand learning, competency-based education, project-based and practice-based teaching, more inclusive and equitable teaching practices, effective use of educational technology, and technology-enabled learning.

It is our hope that this series will be a practical and valuable resource for new and experienced public health educators to support integration of new and exciting topics and approaches into their teaching.

Lisa Sullivan and Sandro Galea

Preface

Welcome to our book!

We want to introduce ourselves and this book by sharing that we love teaching qualitative methods in public health. One reason why we are so enthusiastic about it is that in every course there is at least one student who gets a new sense of the possibilities of what public health research can be—and gets energized. Students love to hear that it is important to prioritize people's lived experiences and that not all data must be reduced to discrete variables. We find that students' energy and enthusiasm revitalizes our own!

Our goal is for this text to be a resource for those who teach qualitative methods in public health—in classrooms that service public health schools and programs as well as out in the field. The primary audience for this book is instructors—not students. We set out to write a book that supports faculty as they prepare to teach the subject, whether for the first time or even if they are a seasoned veteran. We have tried to make sure that this work includes the kinds of content that we, as qualitative researchers, feel is needed in different types of qualitative courses and trainings, and for different types of qualitative students. We've also written with an eye toward what *we* have found we have needed, as teachers of this material. To you, we present our ideas for helping students engage with critical ideas and how we assess those students' understanding of them.

This book is intended to help you address the following questions (as well as many others!):

- How do you describe qualitative methods and analytic approaches to students?

- How do you explain how to operationalize qualitative methods?
- How do you build students' capacity for engaging with qualitative research?
- How do you assess a student's command of qualitative content?
- How do you equip students to read, critique, and contribute to scientific literature using qualitative research methods?

One thing that this book is *not* is a comprehensive qualitative methods coursebook. In fact, during the writing process, we often stopped to remind one another that writing a methods coursebook was not our goal. There is a growing canon of great books for people who want to learn about qualitative methods (see Box 1.5 where we list some of the ones that we have called upon in our teaching careers); you might want to assign or recommend one or more of them for students in your course. Our own work as qualitative researchers and teachers of qualitative methods has benefited from having such resources at hand, and we reference many of these books in our chapters. However, we intend our book to serve as a guide for teaching qualitative methods within public health—hopefully for faculty who already have a pretty good understanding of the field.

We have written with the shared goal of building a public health workforce that has a good grasp of what qualitative methods are, how they should be undertaken, and how the data generated can be used to improve population health. We can't all be qualitative researchers in public health, but it would be wonderful if everyone working in public health were to have a solid understanding of the capacity and limitations of these methods for meeting goals and objectives. Hopefully, our book can play a role in meeting this goal.

This book focuses on helping faculty prepare for classroom-based teaching of qualitative methods in public health. Not all classrooms look alike; we understand that some teaching will be virtual (as is some of ours) and some teaching will be embedded within public health institutions as training rather than a formal credentialed curriculum. We also understand that much learning about qualitative methods is done in an apprentice model, with a student or a group of students learning by *doing outside the classroom*, with input from a more advanced qualitative researcher. If you are embarking on such a mentorship model, there is still likely helpful content here, even if its delivery might look different in such scenarios.

Much of the material we present comes from our own experiences teaching many different qualitative courses, in many formats, at our school that operates on eight-week terms and includes intensive short-course institutes. Over the years, we've worked with so many terrific colleagues and continually evolved our approach to teaching, such that it's all but impossible to keep track of everything we've picked up. We are grateful for the knowledge and experience we've accumulated over the years in collaboration with our colleagues and students. We are indebted to the many faculty who taught qualitative methods at Johns Hopkins before us and to those who teach alongside us now. We are also indebted to every colleague who worked with us developing syllabi, delivering content, grading assignments, providing workshops, and much more. This book is a product and reflection of this collective knowledge.

What to expect from our book

You don't need to read this book from cover to cover, nor do we imagine you progressing through the chapters from beginning to end. We understand that coursebooks don't work like that, and qualitative methods are anything but linear. This book's structure generally mirrors the life of a research project, from thinking of a question to selecting the most appropriate methods to analyzing the data to writing up and disseminating the findings. Its chapters don't, however, have to build on each other. Instead, we intend each one to be useful as a stand-alone for one aspect of teaching. We've also tried to write these chapters such that they can be used to build a coherent, thorough, qualitative curriculum.

In Chapter 1, we provide a foundational overview of how we understand qualitative methods and outline their potential contributions to public health research and practice. This chapter is the "Why?" for this book; the other chapters are more about the "How?" (Two good qualitative question words, as you may note!) In Chapter 2, we present specific issues and important considerations about the nature of your course as you plan course content and begin structuring its educational design. Chapter 3 considers issues related to teaching about the role of theory in qualitative methods, while Chapter 4 engages with *how* to teach qualitative study design. Chapter 5 is especially crucial, as it covers teaching several of the main data collection approaches undertaken in qualitative research (interviews, focus groups, observations, and document analysis), and Chapter 6 tackles the subject of teaching qualitative analysis. In Chapter 7, we discuss how to engage students on important overarching issues, namely ethics, reflexivity, and rigor. Chapter 8 covers the writing and dissemination of qualitative research. Finally, Chapter 9 explores the evaluation of learning and different course-specific assessment approaches. The issue of assessment also runs through many of the chapters in relation to thinking about exercises: both in and out of class, along with individual and group work. In Chapter 10, we bring together a few final observations and well wishes for you as you prepare for the classroom.

While courses are linear, the qualitative research process usually is not. We present these chapters in an order that makes sense to us (and one that mirrors the order in which we often teach). However, you may well want to order your course differently—and that's totally OK! For example, you might want to have students consider how they think differently about rigor for qualitative methods before they've been exposed to specific approaches, whereas we present this material afterward, as a single unit toward the end of this book (in Chapter 7). You may want to put ethical considerations up front or alternatively engage in ethical dialogue once students are familiar with the major data collection approaches. Separating the consideration of data collection methods from analytic strategies might make logical sense or you may feel that waiting to consider data analysis until after talking through data collection methods might result in missing an opportunity to emphasize the importance of engaging analysis concurrently with data collection. We don't think that there is a right or wrong answer to issues of order. However, from our experience, we suggest that you think about the implications of your decisions in terms of how students come to see the various pieces of the methodological puzzle coming together.

In each chapter of this book, we provide materials you are welcome to use in your own course, as well as ideas that you might adapt to make new materials. You'll find some places where we draw the reader's attention to some fundamental information that we label "Qualitative building blocks." We have also included several "Myth busters," in which we call out assumptions that some students come into class with and offer ideas for how you can challenge these. Finally, we include many "Tips and tricks" for teaching a topic or issue in a way that has helped us to deal with a teaching challenge. We also incorporate common student questions and succinct responses that address key concerns without taking you (and your students!) down a rabbit hole.

Our approach to teaching qualitative methods is to center the learner in the process to the greatest extent possible. When teaching something about doing—as qualitative methods is—the delivery of information in readings, lectures, and discussions can only be the beginning (DeLyser, 2008). We agree with Wagner, Kawulich, and Garner's assertion that "experiential learning is one of the most popular approaches to preparing qualitative researchers" (2019, p. 2), as this approach embraces both theoretical concepts and lived experiences. There are many ways to build experiential learning into all kinds of courses and for all kinds of learners, to provide structured opportunities for developing skills, and to learn from inevitable initial missteps. Doing so requires planning, good communication, implementation skills, and the ability to deal positively with students' reactions to emergent issues. At its core, this book features an experiential approach to qualitative teaching and learning.

This is a teaching coursebook for an applied field. We will explore and explain how to teach major topics related to the "why" and "how" of conducting qualitative research in public health. We are aware that our book, like all others, must have boundaries; for this reason, we refrained from including a great deal of information that you may find helpful. We are aware of the many allied approaches often associated with qualitative methods, including photovoice, community-based participatory research, mixed methods, case studies, and ethnography. It has been our experience that these approaches go beyond what can usually be covered in a qualitative methods course in public health and are therefore better served by a stand-alone course. As a result, we decided not to include these approaches in this text.

Audience and terminology

In this book, we use the term "course" to refer to a semester- or quarter-long course. The word "class" and phrase "class session" refer to a single day of the course (usually a one-to-two-hour session). We recognize that there are also occasions when a class on a topic may be independent of a broader course.

We assume that you, the reader, are a faculty member at an institution of higher education. We teach graduate students primarily, including both master's and doctoral-level students. However, many of this book's recommendations would also apply to training people in the public health workforce who are engaged in conducting qualitative research, or undergraduate students. In either case, there may perhaps need to be a few adjustments. For example, undergraduates may not be prepared to do their own independent research but would likely be interested in hands-on research experience that might require more structured support. If you are teaching study teams, colleagues, or other professionals outside of a formal course structure, you may need to make more significant adjustments to the content to ensure that the training is directly applicable to the work being undertaken.

We use the term "students" to refer to the people you teach. We use this term because it is simple and straightforward. We realize that we could have used other terms, such as "learners" or "trainees," with their own connotations, and perhaps in the process give more recognition to the fact that college students, graduate students, and public health workers are adult learners who come into our classrooms with substantial personal and often professional experience. We use "students" to encompass adult learners who are actively constructing their own engagement with material and often bring considerable expertise and understanding developed outside of the classroom. While we may have more specific training in qualitative methods than our students, our role as teachers is to build on students' existing knowledge to guide learning and conversations that engage everyone in the classroom.

Although there is an underlying assumption that we work in a particular professional paradigm with an applied research focus, this book may be useful to readers from other fields, including closely aligned areas such as medicine, nursing, and social work. In contrast, readers from other disciplines—particularly those with rich qualitative traditions themselves, such as sociology or anthropology—may find that some of the assumptions we make about our students and about our professional paradigm do not apply to them.

Owning your course

Ultimately, you will want to own your course. You will need to decide what to teach and how. Our book covers many topics you *could* include in your syllabus and many activities and assignments you *could* consider bringing into your course. But the book is not a prescription: you will need to make choices based on what resonates with your own pedagogical approach and commitments, and your students' needs. Even while writing this book, the four of us found that we did not always immediately agree on context or content. We discussed different approaches and often decided to present alternatives. So, although we have tried to present the material with a unified voice for ease of reading, there are points where members of the authorship team make different choices in our own courses and teaching. We recognize that you may not agree with some of what we say. We may present concepts that you feel are tangential to the core content you want to teach, concepts with which you are not familiar, or concepts you feel uncomfortable teaching because you have not mastered them yourself. We would expect these considerations to factor into how you shape your course. We were motivated to write this book by the hope that you, as readers, will find at least some of the content useful. Whether developing a new course or refreshing one that you've taught for many years, we share the privilege of helping those who are coming behind us realize an expansive view of public health and public health research that qualitative research provides.

Acknowledgments

We are thankful to be part of the Johns Hopkins Bloomberg School of Public Health, an institution that recognized the importance of qualitative methods in public health relatively early and has nurtured support for qualitative methods over the past quarter-century. We have benefitted greatly from the growing community of public health researchers and practitioners who value conducting and teaching qualitative methods within public health. We particularly would like to thank our colleagues who have previously taught or who currently teach qualitative research methods at the Johns Hopkins Bloomberg School of Public Health. Our thoughts in this book have been influenced by the work and ideas of many people inside and outside of the Bloomberg School, including but not limited to Paul Brodwin, Sarah Dalglish, Julie Denison, Robert Dingwall, Joel Gittelsohn, Lance Gravlee, Susan Hannum, Steve Harvey, Lori Leonard, Elli Leontsini, Shannon McMahon, Elizabeth Murphy, Haneefa Saleem, David Seal, Pamela Surkan, Peter Winch, and Amber Wutich.

We also thank the many graduate teaching assistants who helped us provide quality teaching and support for students in many classes over the years. We thank all the individuals who have collaborated with us on syllabus design and discussed creative ideas for how to teach qualitative methods to different students in different formats. We also thank our students—many of whom have become colleagues—for all their insightful questions and course engagement. Over the years, these discussions have refined our pedagogy and deepened our understanding of what qualitative methods can bring to public health.

We owe a deep debt of gratitude to John Brown Spiers, a professional editor whom we engaged partway through our process. John helped us with clarity and harmonize our different voices. We also thank our illustrator, Iulian Thomas (https://www.fiverr.com/weedstation), who took our ideas for images and turned them into stylish and fun aids to our text.

Finally, we thank our families and friends who support us in our personal and professional lives; we could not do what we do without your support. This is true even if they didn't ever really realize that we were writing this book!

Reflexive Statement About the Authorship Team

Four of us wrote this book together. We are similar in many ways, yet we each bring our own unique professional and personal experiences to teaching qualitative research methods in public health. All four of us are PhD-trained, tenured professors at the Johns Hopkins Bloomberg School of Public Health. Two of us completed our doctoral training at the same school where we now teach. The other two completed doctoral training in programs of Anthropology and Sociology, including one of us who trained outside of the United States. All of us are white, cisgender American women. All of us do work that would generally be characterized as more applied than theoretical.

We each focus on different public health topic areas, including cancer control and lived experiences of chronic disease in the United States, health disparities and implementation of public health programs in the United States and Eastern Europe, HIV and sexual health in Africa, and policy implementation to prevent injury and violence in the United States. Each of us identifies primarily as a qualitative researcher and has extensive experience contributing to mixed methods public health research. Between us, we have extensive experience conducting qualitative studies based on qualitative interview data (from open-ended narrative interviews to ethnographic, to semi-structured or structured to key informant). We have conducted studies that draw extensively on focus group data and documents. We have undertaken observational and ethnographic research and have substantial experience publishing work based on analysis of various documents pertinent to public health. Two of us primarily focus on research within the U.S., and two internationally—but all of us have conducted research inside and outside the U.S. None of us identify as a truly community-engaged researcher who fully embodies community-based participatory research practices, although we all attempt to be responsible and ethical research partners. We each engage with the policy process and public health programs somewhat differently.

We are aware that none of us have formal pedagogical training. Rather, we are from a generation (or generations) of academics for whom it was seemingly assumed that one would become a competent educator through a process of osmosis and practice. So, we teach largely the way we ourselves were taught and have informally gained training throughout the years through workshops, readings, and lived experience. In preparing our courses and in the writing of this book, we have been deliberate in considering the learning needs of our students and how we can be prepared to meet their needs in various educational spaces. We teach courses with as few as eight students and as many as 150; we each teach in-person and online. Our courses range from ones that span a semester (two terms) to one-day institute courses, and even more targeted on-site training sessions. We are not perfect teachers, nor do we pretend that our classes are the epitome of teaching qualitative methods in public health. In this book, we share our experiences in the spirit of collaboration and collegiality. We hope that you receive it in that spirit and find it useful!

1
Science and Data

Before we dive into the ins and outs of teaching qualitative methods, it's important to establish a common understanding of why we undertake qualitative research and the theoretical assumptions that underpin this approach. We aim to help students appreciate the place of a qualitative approach within scientific inquiry more broadly. We often call upon the words of Maykut and Morehouse (1994) in our courses by stating that a researcher needs to be able to articulate the reasons for taking a qualitative approach if they are going to be able to "defend the project as a rigorous and valued piece of scholarship" (p. 2). When we teach qualitative methods to public health students, we almost always start by engaging with how most people have been taught to think about science—namely, by introducing two questions:

What are the goals of a scientific study?
What does it look like when science is being done well?

We ask students to think about how researchers determine what is important to know and how they go about seeking answers and invite them to consider what it means to generate knowledge. We start here because we recognize that public health is a field long dominated by a quantitative, objectivist mindset—which is inherently inconsistent with the foundations of qualitative methods. In our courses, we are seeking to "flip the script" in relation to how research might be conducted and why qualitative research is conducted the way that it is.

Teaching Qualitative Research in Public Health. Katherine Clegg Smith et al., Oxford University Press.
© Oxford University Press (2026). DOI: 10.1093/9780197662472.003.0001

For many public health students, a qualitative methods course can be the gateway to an expanded view of science and research (see Figure 1.1). Usually, students have been taught that research is about setting out to find "the truth," and that research should be designed to allow us to get the "right answer" to questions such as, who are the people most likely to experience a health problem or whether a public health intervention really works. For the most part, our students have never been asked to challenge the objectivist view of science, nor have they been invited to critically engage with the underlying assumptions of that view. We routinely ask students to consider whether there are research questions that cannot be answered with a quantitative approach. We also invite them to consider the idea of the world as socially constructed and the legitimacy of multiple authentic perspectives of an event, issue, or scenario. In our classes—and particularly introductory classes—we prioritize referencing the

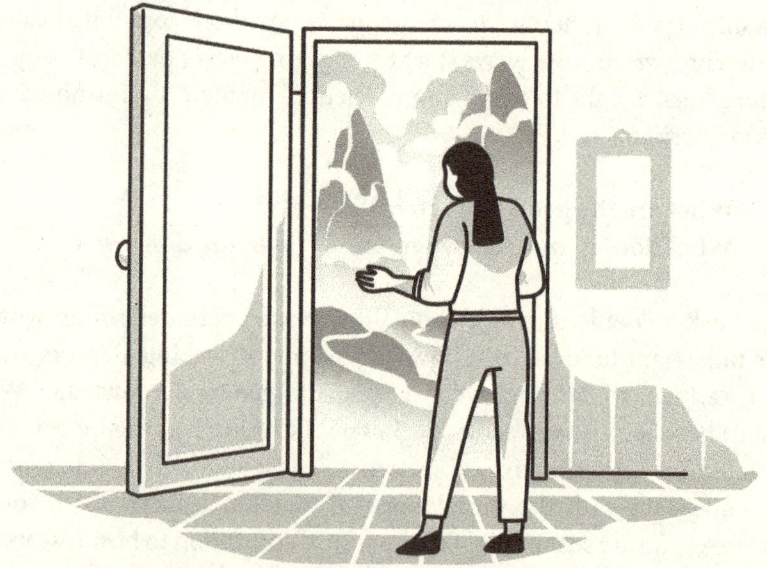

Figure 1.1 Introducing epistemological concepts can expose students to a "new world" of research

philosophy of science and introduce the term "epistemology" (see Chapter 3 for more on this concept).

We find it important to ground our courses in discussions of the nature of the world (ontology) and of how we know and understand the world (epistemology) because doing so allows us to define qualitative methods relative to what they *are* rather than simply describing what they *are not* (e.g., we don't use numbers to determine the importance of a finding; we don't seek population-level generalizability). We also emphasize that some research questions can only be answered through *quantitative* methods, and we set the stage for one of our oft-repeated maxims: the research question should drive the choice of method.

Understanding epistemology helps students reorient their way of thinking such that qualitative methods are understood as an appropriate mechanism for generating useful knowledge. Exposure to epistemology prepares students to engage more fully with the methods, analysis, and work of qualitative research. From the outset of each course, we establish that qualitative methods are built on the recognition that questions can mean different things to different people and on the idea that lived experiences and context can result in different individual truths (Box 1.1). Given this recognition, it makes sense to question whether the pursuit of a single truth (an idea that is so core to common scientific principles) can actually capture the complexity of reality in a way that facilitates full understanding of many public health questions such that they can be addressed. This chapter consists of 10 questions based on discussions we've had with students in class sessions early in our qualitative courses. In addition to establishing a common understanding of key concepts related to qualitative methods, discussions based on these questions can help address misunderstandings and biases that students may bring to the classroom. Such discussions increase the students' receptivity to course readings, class sessions, and assignments. In the process, they maximize their own learning by establishing and building upon a shared foundation of qualitative methods in public health.

Box 1.1 Tips and tricks: Put epistemology up front

Building your qualitative course on an epistemological foundation is one way to frame its content and method and to emphasize what qualitative methods bring to public health. Even with this frame in place, you are likely to encounter some of the tension that crops up in discussions about the use of qualitative methods in public health. Because these methods offer tools to advance the understanding of a topic, they tend to be hypothesis-generating. Public health, though, is action-oriented and seeks answers to inform programs and policies. Creating a learning environment that acknowledges the complementary nature of these different functions, and the historical dominance of quantitative methods, can ease such tension before it dominates the conversation and erodes your ability to meet your learning objectives (see Chapter 3).

What is qualitative research?

It is almost inevitable that on the first day of any qualitative methods course in a public health program, there will be students with either no understanding or a very limited understanding of what is meant by qualitative research. It's also likely that some students will begin the class with an understanding of qualitative methods that could benefit from careful correction or refinement. Wagner et al. (2019) proposed that embarking on qualitative research does not only mean that one is engaging with different research tools or skills, but also that one has a different understanding of the goals of research and how one goes about it. We hold that examining what constitutes a qualitative research study—and what does not— is an important element of any qualitative methods course in public health.

One way to think about this is to ask yourself (and possibly the class) the following questions:

What makes a study qualitative?
What makes a qualitative study valuable?

Qualitative methods embrace a naturalistic approach, meaning that, "we explore issues, ideas, and questions on the ground, in the settings in which they arise, striving to understand and interpret phenomena in terms of the meanings the groups and individuals we study and work with bring to them" (Delyser, 2008, p. 234). Miles and Huberman's (1994) list of characteristics of much "naturalistic" qualitative work is one framework for considering the essential features of a qualitative study (Box 1.2). Introducing each feature with a few empirical examples of exemplary studies may offer insight into what qualitative research is, as well as how it has been applied. Working through examples of model qualitative studies can also help correct any misconceptions about the method.

Box 1.2 Foundational knowledge: Features of qualitative methods

- Qualitative research involves intense and/or prolonged engagement with a given setting or situation.
- Qualitative research prioritizes its participants' perspectives, including both empathetic understanding and bracketing of researchers' preconceptions or assumptions.
- Routinely, qualitative research engages with how people come to understand, account for, act on, and manage everyday situations.
- Qualitative research often minimizes the use of standardized instrumentation, instead prioritizing the researcher as a key instrument for any study.
- Qualitative analysis tends to focus on words and interpretation as the foundation of meaning-making and patterns, rather than quantification to determine what is key.
- Qualitative researchers usually seek a holistic understanding of the phenomenon of study (Miles & Huberman, 1994)

The term "qualitative research" is somewhat heterogeneous and does not necessarily mean the same thing to all people (Hammersley, 2013). When thinking about what makes qualitative research distinct, it can also be helpful to articulate the principles that are either unique to or foundational for qualitative research. Below are some of those principles that we consider elemental. Your list might include others; our list has evolved over time. It may be helpful to share such lists with students, providing opportunities for them to discuss and ask questions. And it may even be the case that, toward the end of the course, the students will want to suggest additional principles based on what they have learned.

Possible principles for qualitative inquiry

- **Qualitative research minimizes the structure imposed by the researcher or the research process.** Researchers tend to go into the real world and prioritize experiences as they occur and words of the people upon whom the research is focused.
- **Qualitative research embraces the complexity of human interactions and social settings rather than trying to control for these.** In qualitative research, we rarely try to select a single variable and determine its relevance to a causal relationship. Rather, qualitative researchers tend to try engaging with many elements of a setting or interaction within their analysis.
- **Qualitative research acknowledges the researcher's inevitable effect on the research process.** Research is a human activity; qualitative research is often centered on human interaction. The data collected and the analyses undertaken therefore reflect the people involved in the research process. This impact is not something to be eliminated (indeed, it isn't possible or desirable to do so). Instead, it is the responsibility of the researcher to acknowledge their impact and understand it as much as possible and present it to the audience for their consideration.

- **Qualitative research is usually best for gathering a deep and detailed understanding of a bounded phenomenon.** The understanding generated from qualitative analysis is often for the purpose of building theory, rather than a broad consideration of a general issue or testing a specific relationship between two or more distinct variables. Explanations and theory-building often motivate qualitative inquiry. The standard is not population-level generalizability.
- **Qualitative research can be helpful for generating explanatory theories.** As outlined above, qualitative research often prioritizes insights generated from data without imposition of a theoretical framework for purposes of hypothesis testing. Theory generation may or may not be followed by more structured theory testing.

Finally, some students may benefit from a comparison of the key features of qualitative and quantitative approaches. Table 1.1 illustrates this type of comparison and draws from comparative elements of different sources. While we try to avoid being reductionist,

Table 1.1 Comparison of key dimensions of qualitative and quantitative approaches

	Qualitative	Quantitative
Design	Emergent	Planned
	Insider's perspective (Emic)	Outsider's perspective (Etic)
	Exploratory	Confirmatory
	Hypothesis-generating	Hypothesis-testing
	Words	Numbers
Methods	Less structured	More structured
	More dynamic/flexible	Less dynamic/flexible
Sampling	Small sample size	Large sample size
	More depth	Less depth
	Purposive	Random
Context	Rich	Less rich
	Multiple factors considered	Individual variable(s) isolated

we recognize that this sort of comparison can be helpful as a starting point, particularly for students who are new to qualitative methods (new students can be advanced doctoral students as well as undergraduates). Students can start to problematize these overly simplistic distinctions later—for example, when they learn that qualitative research can be used to test hypotheses as well as to generate them!

Does qualitative inquiry require a different way of thinking about research?

The field of public health is rooted in an objectivist, biomedical paradigm. At the same time, the field is also inherently multidisciplinary and applied. In the recent past, qualitative research has become recognized as one of the core sets of methods for public health. But teaching qualitative research to people trained largely in an objectivist, biomedical paradigm can create specific challenges. As we will explore in Chapter 3, qualitative research draws from different conceptualizations of how and with what purpose knowledge is generated. It can be difficult to present such conceptualizations of the nature of the world being examined (ontology), and of how we can understand it (epistemology), to students who signed up for a class that they expected would teach them tangible skills right from day one.

Students coming to a qualitative methods class in public health are highly likely to see science as a process of testing hypotheses based on findings from research. The concepts of independence and generalizability are likely important to their understanding of rigorous research design. Also common are student expectations that research processes will lead to the discovery of the truth. Expanding their beliefs such that they can appreciate the role of qualitative methods alongside the established quantitative paradigm is crucial if learners are to also appreciate the role that qualitative methods play in advancing scientific discovery.

We maintain that a level of engagement with ontological and epistemological questions in any qualitative course is a vital part of understanding qualitative methods and how they contribute to meeting public health goals. This engagement is also a helpful means of avoiding "methodolatry," whereby students idolize methods in an uncritical, postpositivistic approach and are unfamiliar with the distinct epistemological and critical foundations of fields such as qualitative research and health equity work (Bowleg, 2017). We will also discuss when it might not be essential to use terms like "epistemology" and "ontology," which are potentially unfamiliar and abrasive for some students, when talking about foundational issues in qualitative methods.

Is qualitative inquiry science?

Whether qualitative inquiry constitutes science depends largely on how we define "science." The term is often equated with the concept of methodological rigor and a mode of inquiry based on an objectivist positionality (Pelto & Pelto, 1978). Qualitative research should be rigorous—often, though, it is not conducted from an objectivist perspective. Does this therefore mean that qualitative research isn't science?

Well, for one thing, defining science around objectivistic enquiry is a narrow definition of science (Pelto & Pelto, 1978): it precludes consideration of the accidents and chance circumstances that generate new research ideas or produce insights into a phenomenon. Moreover, many scientific fields (biology, geology, astronomy) center particularistic and historical inquiry and produce different canons of evidence, rather than those derived from controlled experiments. Based on this understanding of how knowledge is produced, Pelto and Pelto offered a broader definition:

"[Science is] the structure and process of discovery and verification of systematic and reliable knowledge about any relatively enduring aspect of the universe, carried out by means of empirical observation, and the development of concepts and propositions for interrelating and explaining such observations."

(Pelto & Pelto, 1978, p. 22)

Following this definition, we proceed based on the belief that qualitative approaches are very much science and part of the scientific endeavor, with rules, techniques, and principles that have been refined over years and across fields—among them public health.

What are the scholarly origins of qualitative research?

In teaching the foundations of qualitative research, you might feel it is important to raise awareness that although these approaches may be new or novel methods for public health, they have long histories and traditions in the social science disciplines of anthropology and sociology, as well as in the humanities disciplines of cultural studies, history, and linguistics. Fields such as biology and animal ecology also have fieldwork and empirical observation at their core. Discussing qualitative studies' contributions to these fields, and, in turn, contributions to how we understand social structure and human behavior, can be illuminating.

The history of qualitative methods in fields such as sociology and anthropology reaches back to these disciplines' foundations and founders. Both have long prioritized immersive fieldwork, participant observation, and conversational interviews to understand the complex nature of human societies and social institutions. Pioneers such as Bronisław Malinowski and Franz Boas in anthropology and Howard Becker and Robert Park in sociology championed qualitative approaches in the early 20th century, each emphasizing the importance of spending extended time with the people they studied and learning their cultural practices, beliefs, and socially constructed meanings. Over the years, qualitative methods in these disciplines have evolved and diversified, incorporating techniques such as ethnographic surveys, focus groups, life histories, textual analysis, and archival research.

The history of qualitative methods in public health is a testament to the recognition of the multifaceted, context-dependent nature of health and well-being. While public health traditionally relied on quantitative approaches to measure and assess health outcomes, the incorporation of qualitative methods has provided a deeper understanding of the social, cultural, and behavioral factors that shape health disparities and health-seeking behaviors. Over time, qualitative methods gained a steady foothold in public health research, facilitating the exploration of complex issues like health beliefs, patient experiences, healthcare access, and community dynamics. By centering the lived experiences and social contexts that influence health, qualitative methods have contributed to more comprehensive and patient-centered approaches to public health interventions and policies. In Box 1.3, we provide guidance on how an instructor can introduce the well-established history of qualitative methods in social science disciplines, as well as ongoing resistance to these methods in some areas of clinical and public health scholarship.

Box 1.3 Tips and tricks: Qualitative methods in aligned academic disciplines

Qualitative methods have a rich history in a range of academic disciplines that inform public health (e.g., sociology, anthropology, nursing, social work, humanities). In order to help students consider and appreciate these origins, you might ask students to do the following:

- Identify key qualitative researchers from their home disciplines.
- Discuss these qualitative researchers' major contributions to the field.

continued

Box 1.3 *continued*

For an additional discussion point, have students read and discuss the *British Medical Journal*'s 2016 decision to no longer publish qualitative research, along with the response, from Greenhalgh et al., that argued for the value of qualitative methods and the contributions qualitative perspectives have made to medicine and public health.

Declaration: https://www.doi.org/10.1136/bmj.i641 (Loder et al., 2016)

Response: https://www.doi.org/10.1136/bmj.i563 (Greenhalgh et al., 2016)

Returning to the present, you also might provide students with a selected qualitative journal article (or two) on a topic that you know is pertinent to some or all of the students in the course, or ask students to do a simple search for current qualitative research studies in their areas of interest, and discuss the contributions of this work with a partner. At a more basic level, students could be asked to submit three or four citations of qualitative work on a particular topic as a homework exercise.

We reference anthropology as one disciplinary source of the qualitative tools used by public health researchers. Qualitative methods are often used to provide detailed exploratory and explanatory accounts of social phenomena and experiences. The embedded style of anthropological fieldwork that requires yearslong engagement on the part of researchers provides useful context but is different from the approach to fieldwork reported in public health journals. In public health, we tend to rely more on short site visits, local collaborators, and sustained engagement with a research topic or area over long periods of time, rather than an immersive field experience that lasts six or more months (a study duration typical of anthropology and ethnography). One foundation of qualitative education in public health is a balance between the philosophical foundations of qualitative methods and the practical need for these methods in an applied discipline.

In addition to introducing students to the longstanding disciplinary roots of qualitative research, we feel it is also important to acknowledge that public health research is distinct from many of these fields in some fundamental ways. The goal of social sciences research is often to examine or understand a topic without the expectation that the research team will either intervene or seek to make change. In contrast, public health is an applied discipline in which research typically has the stated goal of improving health and well-being. For example, a common need in public health is quick data generation to inform the response to a pressing health issue. As a result, the qualitative methods we use in public health are sometimes adapted or otherwise different from those used in the social sciences. It's often critical for public health researchers to consider the interventional applications of qualitative findings. How will policymakers, community leaders, and others understand your work? How will they use it to make meaningful change? How might their use shape the data you collect and the analysis you undertake? The intended application can shape the data collection undertaken and the analysis and dissemination approach.

What is the role of theory in qualitative research?

Much qualitative research is not intended to engage in "theory testing." This is not to say, however, that theory is tangential to our work. Qualitative research really shines when attention is paid to both theory and data throughout the research process. Moving beyond thin, description-only analyses detached from the existing literature means acknowledging that theory—including social science and biomedical theory—helps ground and enrich the practice of qualitative methods and influences the meaning of the data we collect. Of course, there are some research questions that seek only descriptive results, for example, when there are significant gaps in the literature around the general contours of a specific phenomenon. But we caution against coming into the classroom with *only* this orientation. Instead, we encourage faculty to engage your students in assessing when descriptive findings are the goal and when theoretical considerations would provide a richer set of findings and more informed analyses. Chapter 3 provides a detailed consideration of teaching theory and qualitative methods.

Are qualitative methods a standard part of public health training?

The Council on Education for Public Health (CEPH) includes qualitative methods among its Evidence-Based Approaches to Public Health Competencies and offers guidance for how to fit qualitative methods within the full suite of competencies for professional degree programs. CEPH accreditation requires schools and programs of public health to demonstrate an offering of courses that meet each foundational competency identified for the field, including how to select, analyze, and interpret qualitative and quantitative data in response to specific public health needs. The inclusion of qualitative methods among the field's foundational competencies tracks with the increasing interest in and use of qualitative methods we have observed throughout our careers.

As such, instructors of qualitative methods at an accredited school of public health or affiliated with an accredited public health program may find great interest in and support for these methods but can also face significant headwinds. Students and faculty often express their appreciation for qualitative research's ability to capture participants' voices and highlight lived experience in stories that incorporate the broader social and economic forces central to public health. However, while the infrastructure that supports quantitative approaches is well established in most schools (some with entire departments of biostatistics and epidemiology), departments devoted to qualitative methods are absent. Qualitative approaches are also less likely to be diffused throughout the curriculum alongside quantitative approaches and perspectives. As a result, students may enroll in qualitative methods and research design courses with a limited vocabulary and set of expectations about what constitutes qualitative data and how to operational-ize concepts such as rigor and validity, or other scientific princi-ples, in ways that are not embedded in a quantitative, objectivist epistemology.

On that note, students may also come to class under the assump-tion that qualitative methods are easy and that anyone can do qual-itative research—without much training or any at all. Furthermore, there is a tendency among students to dismiss qualitative methods as a simple summary of opinions on a given topic, or as an enterprise more journalistic than scientific. Regardless of any preconceived notions, students likely have little background in either the course content or concepts about the scientific method. If they are to under-stand and appreciate qualitative methods, you may need to guide them in a re-examination of some basic assumptions about scientific inquiry.

Teaching a qualitative methods course in a school or program of public health can therefore be both a highly rewarding and very demanding task. The benefits can be extraordinary: your stu-dents may take giant leaps forward in their knowledge, which is tremendously exciting for both them and their instructor! And the drawbacks can be just as taxing: it is of course possible that students will come to class entrenched in an objectivist mindset and unprepared—perhaps even unwilling—to consider alternative ways of conceptualizing knowledge and science. One purpose of this book is therefore to maximize the potential for great rewards when helping students up a steep learning curve while minimiz-ing any pushback from students who have trouble breaking free of quantitative paradigms (Box 1.4).

> **Box 1.4 Tips and tricks: Engaging with students steeped in an objectivist approach**
>
> Some students may come to your course with some skepticism about qualitative methods and an assumption that there is an inherent superiority of an objectivist epistemology. Anticipating that you may encounter these students can be helpful. With a willingness to discuss, you can help students understand that qualitative methods are legitimate, have a long and robust history, and make important contributions to public health. We have had students tell us that this was one of the most unexpected and important insights gained during their qualitative training.

In the following chapters, we will explore the foundations of qualitative research and teach specific methods and analytical approaches. It is essential that students in a qualitative methods course learn about these methods' origins, what the methods are designed to achieve, and how public health researchers are developing the methods to meet our disciplinary needs. This is not always what students expect or think they need from a methods course, as such an approach may not be the shortest path to the skills they seek. In our experience, faculty need to help students understand why to use qualitative methods and the potential important public health impact that these methods can have—alongside the important "how to" elements of the course.

What is the role of qualitative research in public health and what are the venues in which it is conducted?

We often think of public health first in relation to identifying population-wide patterns of disease. Indeed, this work is an important first step for developing interventions that prevent or address ill health in large numbers. However, if this is the work of public health, then what role is there for qualitative research? The reality of public health is much more complex, and qualitative research has a role to play in addressing almost any public health problem. For example:

- Qualitative methods can be used to comprehend why a condition becomes a policy priority—or why it does not (e.g., Shawar & Shiffman, 2020).
- Qualitative methods are useful tools for understanding how a community views a problem (e.g., Smythe et al., 2022).
- Qualitative methods help us appreciate the experience of living with or undergoing treatment for a condition (e.g., Othman et al., 2022).
- Qualitative research can be instrumental in teaching us how a disease spreads and about the public health response (Taylor et al., 2018).
- Qualitative methods are a critical tool for examinations of why interventions may or may not be effective (Wynters et al., 2021).

How do qualitative and quantitative methods work together?

Methodologists are often passionate about how they conduct research. Miles and Huberman (1994) were audacious enough to describe qualitative data as "sexy" because they allow researchers rich insights into local contexts and how events relate to one another. This passion can sometimes lead people into the habit of thinking and talking about how their way is "better" than other means of learning about the world. In fact, it's not unusual for qualitative researchers to dismiss the contributions or the validity of quantitative research, and vice versa. We don't find it helpful to construct and defend alternative methodological camps—certainly not for a field as complex and applied as public health.

Instead, we suggest that as educators it is our job to build a foundation for qualitative methods training among public health students that doesn't pit qualitative and quantitative research against one another. Rather, we present a framework of methods as complementary tools. While qualitative and quantitative research do come from different ontological and epistemological perspectives (see Chapter 3), this does not mean that they are incompatible.

A presentation of the ways that qualitative and quantitative work complement each other could consider the role of each type of research in relation to the following.

Different stages of knowledge production

An introduction to qualitative research can be set within the presentation of a cyclical research process that includes exploration, examination, and explanation; qualitative methods can be applied to each stage of this process. It is common to find studies that begin an inquiry with qualitative methods to explore the nature of a phenomenon and facilitate further examination (either qualitatively or quantitatively). Qualitative studies can also help examine a process with follow-on explanatory stages that are qualitative or quantitative. Finally, targeted, qualitative explanatory work is often quite useful as a follow-on from unexpected or hard to understand quantitative results.

Different types of research questions

Another way to present the complementary nature of qualitative and quantitative research and to ground consideration of qualitative research's value to public health is to consider how each methodology relates to the different types of research questions. Qualitative research can be particularly powerful for answering "How" questions related to process, "What" questions that serve to describe, and "Why" questions that generate understanding of context and motivation. Often, we ask students to consider whether "Who," "When," and "Where" questions are ever best answered qualitatively. In this context, we suggest that the above are the kinds of questions that are usually best addressed through quantification. It can be helpful to convey the importance of both methodological approaches by showing how each one may be particularly useful in relation to a specific type of question.

Different types of information

Consider also the different types of information that qualitative and quantitative research produce. For whom is the research intended and what are the ways in which it can be useful? For example, Patton argues that outcome evaluations that incorporate client stories—of interactions with staff, experiences with programs, personal growth, and changes in response to programs—can provide a richness that numbers alone cannot (Patton, 2002, p. 153).

What is the role of the qualitative researcher?

Qualitative methods might challenge students' thinking about how they conceptualize the researcher's role. More than likely, your students will have been trained to believe that good research means minimizing or outright eliminating the researcher's influence on the process or the data generated. They may have a clear sense that all researchers should strive for objectivity, the elimination of bias, and the creation of conditions that allow for the replication of processes and findings. A good course in qualitative research, though, will likely call all of this into question.

Qualitative research tends to draw upon a constructivist paradigm (see Chapter 3) that considers the researcher as key to the construction of the research process, the data collected, and the analyses undertaken. This paradigm presents research as an interactive and human process. It is therefore not possible to remove who the researcher is or how they relate to their subject of study from the study itself. The researcher is the instrument of data collection, which means that researchers should be aware of their capacity to shape their research and the data it generates. A researcher's identifying characteristics are also likely to influence how findings are interpreted and possibly whether and how they are utilized to make change. Instead of objectivity, qualitative researchers therefore tend to highlight the notions of reflexivity and reflexive practices. In our courses, we seek to teach students how to avoid the trap of thinking that only one kind of researcher can conduct a particular type of research with a specific community. We talk instead about how to embrace the importance of perspective in qualitative research and mechanisms for examining the perspective(s) of the researcher and participants (see Chapter 7).

What is the best way to learn about qualitative methods?

Many students come to our qualitative courses fervent in their desire to become skilled enough in qualitative research to start taking on their own projects as quickly as possible. Doctoral students regularly enter the classroom with an idea for a dissertation aim (or two or three) that they feel would be best addressed by a qualitative approach. Master's students often find that qualitative methods training is important for a field placement or job opportunity. Increasingly, a demonstration of qualitative skills can be an important part of their public health résumé. Students engaged in on-site methods training almost always have a specific application—possibly work that is due to start immediately or is even possibly underway! The overarching wish is usually to come away from a qualitative course with a readiness to conduct real research tasks.

Nonetheless, it can be challenging to give students opportunities for fieldwork or experiential learning in every qualitative course. It is important for course learning objectives to be clear to all at the outset. It may be that the goal of a course is for students to learn about qualitative methods and take on actual research tasks during the course. Alternatively, there may be an opportunity for students to practice the skills needed for qualitative research (such as observation or interviewing) without integrating this into actual research. There are also situations where the course's scope is such that it is preferable to expose students to qualitative work that is done well, rather than emphasizing that they should engage in learning to "do" qualitative research as part of the course. In an introductory course with students who have little prior exposure to qualitative interviewing, for example, they may learn at least as much from studying existing interviews than from conducting their own. There also may simply be too little time or too few resources for you, as faculty, to facilitate such opportunities. This is particularly true with large classes. It may also be more appropriate (and valuable) for students to gain experience by joining a research team as a junior member and learning through an apprenticeship model.

Not all students in a qualitative course will want or need to gain hands-on experience in conducting qualitative research—but many will be seeking this. It is not unusual for us to enhance the often limited "hands on" elements of our courses by explicitly calling upon our own lived experiences as researchers in the classroom, sharing with the students our instruments and data (as much as possible), and the articles and reports that we've written—to give them a realistic sense of what qualitative research is like. In our foundational qualitative courses, we also emphasize the importance of being an informed *consumer* of qualitative research and the value of explicit training to be such a consumer. In terms of being a consumer of qualitative methods, we recognize that faculty are also consumers. In Box 1.5, we provide a nonexhaustive list of qualitative methods texts that we have found to be particularly useful in planning for and delivering various qualitative methods courses in public health.

Box 1.5 Foundational knowledge: Qualitative texts that we have found to be useful

---

If you are looking for grounding in qualitative methods or approaches with which you are less familiar, these are potentially good places to start for an overview of qualitative methods and/or analysis. There are also many other resources in the reference list of this book.

continued

Box 1.5 *continued*

- Braun, V., & Clarke, V. (2021). *Thematic analysis: A practical guide*. Sage Publications.
- Green, J., & Thorogood, N. (2004). *Qualitative methods for health research*. Sage Publications.
- Janesick, V. J. (2016). *"Stretching" exercises for qualitative researchers* (4th ed.). Sage Publications.
- Maykut & Morehouse. (1994). *Beginning qualitative research: A philosophical and practical guide*. Routledge.
- Miles, M., Huberman, A., & Saldaña, S. (2019). *Qualitative data analysis: A methods sourcebook* (4th ed.). Sage Publications.
- Patton, M. Q. (2002). *Qualitative research & evaluation methods* (3rd ed.). Sage Publications.
- Saldaña, J. (2015). *The coding manual for qualitative researchers* (3rd ed.). Sage Publications.
- Silverman, D. (2011). *Interpreting qualitative data*. Sage Publications.
- Silverman, D., & Marvasti, A. (2008). *Doing qualitative research: A comprehensive guide*. Sage Publications.
- Timmermans, S., & Tavory, I. (2022). *Data analysis in qualitative research: Theorizing with abductive analysis*. University of Chicago Press.

Summary

Qualitative methods are important components of the research toolbox available for answering pressing public health questions. In order to make use of these tools, it is important to know what they are and where they come from. Engaging students with these issues will necessitate a consideration of the worldview and philosophy of science that informs how qualitative researchers learn about the world and generate knowledge. As a teacher, reflecting on these fundamental relationships can help you think more deeply about what you teach your students and how that material will in turn influence your students' overall growth as public health professionals.

2
Considerations in Course Design

What do we train people to do?

In public health, we train students for different qualitative research roles. At a foundational level, students may be consumers of qualitative studies, commissioners/funders of qualitative research, staff or faculty supporting qualitative projects, or investigators who want to undertake their own qualitative studies. These students might wish to enhance their work as practitioners who do a little qualitative research as part of a broad portfolio or they may be preparing to become fully-fledged qualitative researchers.

In our experience, public health programs do not usually have the capacity to stratify their students into homogeneous groups for methods training (for example, through a progressive and cumulative curriculum with introductory, intermediate, and advanced qualitative methods courses). However, this kind of stratification would make designing any individual course a little easier! At our school, we commonly have students of different skill and knowledge levels in the same classroom (be it in person or online) and with very different foundational knowledge and learning goals sitting side by side. Regardless of the situation in your courses, we have tips and considerations for both embarking on a new course and revisiting a well-established one. Barraket (2005, p. 2) identified an integration of student-centered learning and traditional methods as being a "recipe for success" with diverse research methods audiences.

Teaching Qualitative Research in Public Health. Katherine Clegg Smith et al., Oxford University Press.
© Oxford University Press (2026). DOI: 10.1093/9780197662472.003.0002

A learner-centered approach

We believe that education should place the student at the core of all aspects of its design. To this end, we address student considerations *before* we come to faculty considerations. A student-centered course will deemphasize a didactic transfer of technical information about how qualitative data are collected and analyzed, instead prioritizing engagement with what we can learn from those who came before us and how we can apply that knowledge to the imagining and conducting of our qualitative studies. Instructors who embrace a learner-centered approach will also create opportunities for experiential learning, active reflexive consideration, and peer modeling. Barraket (2005) has suggested a "holistic" model of methods teaching, one that also includes space for peer engagement alongside the didactic conferral of crucial information when necessary.

In addition to these student-centered methods, we use much of our own research experience, along with a storytelling style, to convey the realities and complexities of qualitative public health research. Incorporating your own experiences into the classroom and being honest with students about processes, outcomes, and decision-making—both right and wrong—can help them understand how what they learn in the classroom translates into the real world and also understand that there is rarely one correct way to design, implement, and evaluate a study.

Identifying students' needs for the course

As previously discussed, qualitative methods' end uses for public health students are quite varied. Bloom's taxonomy (1956) can be a useful framework for conceptualizing different learning objectives and a helpful anchor when designing your course objectives. The taxonomy is also adopted by the Council on Education for Public Health (CEPH), the public health accrediting body in the United States, which can make it a particularly useful reference when designing a course for eventual accreditation review.

We see at least one important area of distinction that can be useful for structuring a course:

> **Is it your goal that, upon completion of the course, your students gain literacy in qualitative methods? Or is it that your students have expertise in qualitative methods?**

Another way to think about this is:

> **Do you want to train your students to be skilled consumers of qualitative research or to undertake qualitative research themselves?**

This prompt is foundational for developing any course's learning objectives and associated assessments. It is important that you decide whether you want to prepare your students to engage with qualitative methods critically or to undertake their own research—and that you communicate your intent to your students. Ultimately, you need to know where you want to take students on their learning journey so you can plan a route that best serves the students' needs and is consistent with your educational capacity (Figure 2.1) If your students are primarily laboratory scientists or statisticians (and in some of our classes, this is the case), it may be sufficient for them to have a general sense that qualitative research exists and is one of many ways in which public health problems can be understood. For a PhD student with a qualitative dissertation aim in mind, or a public health specialist engaging in training related to a specific, commissioned project, the need is quite different.

To be considered qualitatively literate, students need to have a good answer to the following two questions:

> **What are qualitative methods?**
> **Why are qualitative methods important for reaching public health goals?**

Both questions are key to one's own qualitative work and to the capacity for assessing whether qualitative research that one encounters is rigorous and worth attending to.

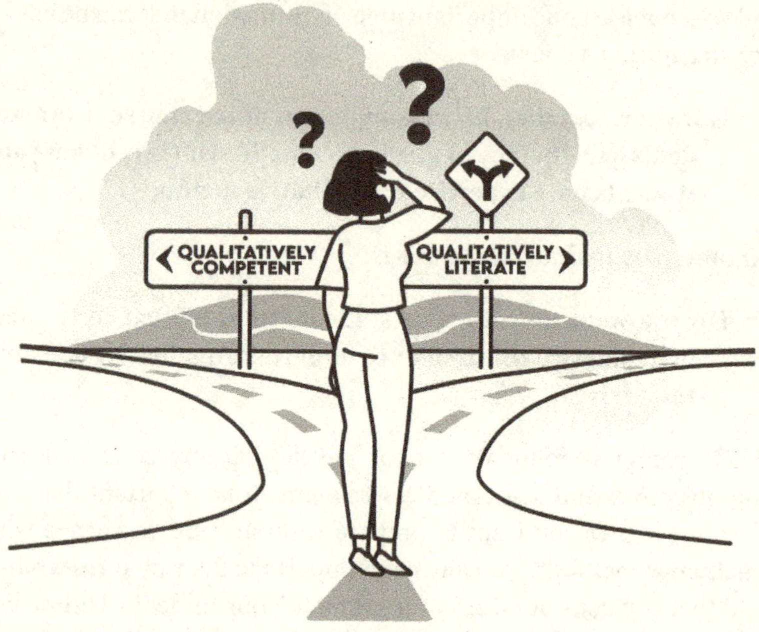

Figure 2.1 Qualitative courses can be designed with different endpoints in mind

In many instances, students will enter a qualitative course classroom wanting and needing to go beyond foundational qualitative literacy. For slightly more intensive classes, your goal may be to have students (be they undergraduates, master's, or doctoral students) understand what qualitative research is, be able to describe the main qualitative data collection methods, and understand why one might select one method over another to achieve research goals. These medium-intensity classes may be for "consumers" of qualitative research who may someday work on multidisciplinary research teams or evaluate research articles in peer-reviewed publications, but who do not plan to be leading qualitative research themselves. If you design your class to introduce concepts but not focus on skill-building, a practitioner who wants hands-on interview training may not find it a good fit. It is better, for both them and you, that the student identifies such a disconnect based on the course description or syllabus rather than finding themselves frustrated with a course that does not provide the skill-building they sought. On the other hand, the intensity of a course that will prepare students to embark on their own qualitative study may be too much for a student who is seeking to be an informed consumer of research that uses qualitative methods but has little or no intention of conducting their own qualitative work.

When designing your course and its assessments, consider how both you and your students will know whether they have accomplished the course goals. One way to determine this is with a backward design approach to articulating course goals and objectives, followed by assessments and instructional and experiential opportunities/exposures.

Course design, learning objectives, and accreditation considerations

"Backward design" or "backward planning" (McTighe & Wiggins, 2012) is a curriculum design approach that involves designing educational experiences by first identifying desired learning outcomes or goals and then determining the instructional activities and assessments that will help students achieve those goals. The backward design process typically consists of three stages:

1. **Identify learning outcomes**. Define the learning outcomes or essential understandings you want students to achieve. These outcomes should be specific, measurable, and aligned with educational standards or objectives.

2. **Determine acceptable evidence**. Once you've established your desired outcomes, consider the evidence or assessment that will demonstrate whether students have achieved those outcomes. This could include tests, projects, presentations, or other measures.

3. **Plan learning experiences and instruction**. With your outcomes and assessments in mind, plan the instructional activities, lessons, and experiences that will best support your students' learning. This involves selecting appropriate instructional strategies, resources, and materials to facilitate student understanding and engagement.

The backward design approach emphasizes that teaching and learning should be purposeful and goal oriented. Starting from your end goals can help ensure that your instructional practices align with your desired outcomes and that your students will be engaged in meaningful learning experiences. It can also help focus your instruction on essential knowledge and skills, promote deeper understanding, and encourage the transfer of learning to real-world contexts. In Box 2.1, we provide the learning objectives for three of our courses that have distinct student audiences, goals, and formats.

Box 2.1 Tips and tricks: Learning objectives for three different qualitative courses

---

Listed below are the learning objectives for our foundational qualitative course on establishing qualitative literacy. We explicitly do **not** attempt to prepare students in this course to conduct their own qualitative research, and we communicate this clearly in the learning objectives for this two-credit, eight-week course.

Upon successful completion of this course, students will be able to do the following:

- explain the basic concepts of iterative design, purposive sampling, and reflexivity
- distinguish between objectivist and constructivist epistemologies
- provide examples of the different types of qualitative data that appear in public health studies
- identify whether qualitative or quantitative methods are best suited for a given research question

- describe key features of study quality (rigor) for qualitative studies
- examine and contrast different approaches to qualitative data analysis
- describe the ways in which qualitative research is incorporated into research projects

Contrast these learning objectives with those from a more advanced and targeted three-credit analysis course, one that introduces, develops, and provides opportunities to practice analytical skills. It is our expectation that, by the end of this more advanced course, students will have the capacity to perform qualitative analysis tasks on their own—with faculty support (as is appropriate for all student projects).

Upon successful completion of this course, students will be able to do the following:

- explain the relationship between qualitative research questions, data collection, analytic method, and interpretative approach
- distinguish different qualitative analytic traditions
- conceptualize the role of the researcher in data analysis and interpretation
- justify a decision regarding use (or not) of a qualitative analysis software package
- develop and apply a coding framework to qualitative data
- evaluate the quality and rigor of published qualitative research
- explain how data collection, transformation, and management processes affect data analysis and interpretation

Note that many of these course objectives include understanding the "whys" of qualitative methods and being an informed consumer of qualitative research, in addition to the skill-oriented objectives that signal more advanced learning goals. In our experience, these foundational components are worth revisiting in most, if not all, qualitative courses.

Finally, below are the learning objectives for a condensed-format, one-credit class, intended for students and practitioners at all levels, on the

continued

Box 2.1 *continued*

---

use of qualitative data analysis software programs. This course is akin to an on-site training that one might do with public health practitioners who need specific skills related to ongoing work. These objectives are intended to transmit the practical skills needed to use qualitative software packages in current or planned data analysis—students want to leave this course ready to work!

Upon successful completion of this course, students will be able to do the following:

- identify the benefits and drawbacks of using computer-assisted qualitative data analysis and defend a decision to use a specific qualitative data analysis software program (or not)
- use software throughout a research project, from data collection through analysis
- use computer-assisted qualitative data analysis software (CAQDAS) to import, query, and manipulate qualitative data
- identify the appropriate data analysis features within a CAQDAS program to answer a particular type of research question or data query

Course structure considerations

Course length and credit hours

Whether a course extends over an entire semester (typically 16 weeks), a quarter (eight weeks), or an intensive interim session (a few days or weeks), the number of credits and mix of in-class contact hours and "homework" hours are important factors when you are considering the depth and breadth of material you can realistically cover. The same principle applies to a noncredit training session that one might be asked to design for public health practitioners. Given the tendency to be overly optimistic about what "realistically" means, we find it helpful to start planning for a new course by thinking about the number of weeks, classes, and contact hours that make up the course and, from there, mapping out, as reasonably as possible, what we will be able to teach in the time that we have. We believe a realistic accounting of the extent to which we can teach both the "why" and the "how," as well as the appropriate level of content exposure for the students, will contribute to course success.

Courses as part of a curriculum

In addition to considering how much you can accomplish in a single course, it is also important that you evaluate each course within the broader curriculum to which students are exposed. Whether your students' training involves other qualitatively oriented classes or is primarily quantitative, for example, will help you decide whether your qualitative methods course is best focused on exposure to concepts or mastery of skills. Also, some degree programs have relatively set curricula in which all students mostly take the same classes; others allow for more individually tailored study. The extent to which students in your course share a coherent set of foundational concepts, theoretical orientations, or training goals will influence the amount of class time you should dedicate to establishing a common language and approach before delving into more specific methodological or analytic aspects. Similarly (and as outlined in Chapter 5), students in public health often come to methods classes having been exposed to a broad range of discipline-specific theoretical frameworks, including psychology, sociology, and economics. These diverse backgrounds may make it challenging for you to establish a unifying perspective or common approach for students to understand the philosophical and epistemological foundations of qualitative approaches and goals of qualitative inquiry—especially if you are teaching a short or intensive course. Nevertheless, in our experience, spending some time learning about your students' starting points is always helpful. Likewise, it is also important to consider where the course is situated in terms of sequence—how a course relates to other courses and the overall structure of the educational program. It involves considering the course's objectives, content, and learning outcomes in relation to the larger educational goals. A course in advanced qualitative methods should be designed with an understanding of the foundational courses that precede it, as well as the more specialized courses that will follow, to ensure that students have a coherent learning experience where each course builds upon the previous one, reinforcing and expanding knowledge. Similarly, educational programs often follow a progression, from introductory courses to more advanced ones. The course may require prior knowledge or skills from earlier courses, which impacts how well students are prepared.

Teaching modalities

The expansion and increased accessibility of video conferencing and online course management platforms have created new possibilities for course formats and audiences. A decade ago, we couldn't have imagined that we would be able to teach an online, asynchronous class to nearly 200 students at a time—but we've now done exactly this, and we are constantly working to improve our capacity as educators in an online space. And there are some real advantages to this option. Online classes enable students who are unable to meet in the same physical space to interact with and learn from each other. They allow students who otherwise couldn't afford the money or the time to enroll in courses and engage with faculty and their peers. Students in an online class may have more diverse backgrounds and a wider range of goals than those in traditional in-person courses. Conceivably, students in a single course could be a mix of traditional degree-seeking students, public health practitioners and policy makers, and field staff who need specific training. This should be a consideration in online course design.

The course structure and modality of delivery both have implications for how students interact with the instructor and each other and how they engage with course material. Whatever the format, it is our experience that students usually learn best through hands-on involvement and active engagement with instructors and other learners. Asynchronous or online classes may limit opportunities for such engagement—which may, in turn, require you to radically rethink your teaching strategies. If an online class enrolls hundreds of students, for example, you will need to consider how you can meet their learning needs in a way that is consistent with the course goals and pedagogical principles.

We have found that we can cover all the same didactic content online that we can in our in-person courses and make the sessions engaging and interactive. However, converting hands-on, project-based learning to an online format requires a willingness to adapt and be creative (Box 2.2). For example, because students in online classes may be spread across different time zones and even different countries, the practicalities of group-based, qualitative projects in the real world—Institutional Review Board (IRB) review and ensuring the ethical conduct of participant interactions, to give just two examples—may become nearly impossible. However, we are mindful that this is likely to change as online interactions become more common, and we would love to learn from others who may have found ways to address these challenges.

Box 2.2 Tips and tricks: Cultivating a positive asynchronous online course

- Incorporate opportunities for regular live (synchronous) touch points for students who are looking for this as part of their learning.
- Prioritize an active discussion forum to facilitate peer exchange and learning. This probably means making discussion board posts part of student assessment, as well as active engagement with the forum content by the faculty member and/or teaching assistant (TA).
- Think hard before introducing group work. For students who do not share physical space and may not be in the same time zone,

continued

Box 2.2 *continued*

---

group work can be a real challenge. Should you include group work, make sure all students understand its value for the course and themselves, and provide structures to help groups succeed. Timelines for product generation and delineation of group member roles can be helpful.

- We find it highly beneficial to have two instructors (including possibly a TA) present at any synchronous online session: one can focus on class structure—content delivery and/or setting up activities—while the second handles all technical aspects: monitoring chats, handling breakout rooms, and so on.
- It is helpful to set your expectations for the students' use of video in synchronous sessions. It can be very challenging to run an engaging session when most students have their cameras turned off.
- Whenever possible, use the tools that help make interactive, engaged learning: chat, breakout rooms, polling, and whiteboards, among others.
- At the end of each class, have students engage in an interactive exercise. For example, students might write a reflective paragraph on who they are and how their identity affects their research. They might engage with a partner in crafting a discussion board post related to a topic raised in class. Another idea would be to assign an exercise comparing deductive and open coding.

Getting hands-on experience with data collection and analysis

One key decision you need to make in designing your qualitative methods course is the extent to which the students will get real-life or hands-on experience collecting and analyzing data. Will your course be self-contained, or will your students interact with the world outside the classroom? Some of our courses are entirely didactic, based solely on readings, lectures, and interactions between student and instructor. We also teach classes in which students conduct interviews with people other than their fellow students and conduct observations in public settings. Most researchers would probably agree that there is no better training than experiential learning. You can only learn so much about what it is like to observe and take field notes or interview from someone else's description—you get so much more out of trying it out for yourself! At the same time, it isn't always going to be possible to get all students "out in the field," nor is this necessary to meet every course's learning goals. So, it is important to think about why "hands-on" learning is being prioritized as well as how it is best done.

In our view, there are five primary ways to approach hands-on experience with research in any course structure. However, you may well come up with an alternative that combines some of these—or is something altogether different.

1. **No hands-on experience.** Not all courses will have the time or capacity to include hands-on activities—and, if the learning objectives for your course focus more on gaining qualitative literacy than readiness to do qualitative research, this is not a problem. In such a course, students can learn from examples: videos of interviews or focus groups, or a documentary that may work as an observation proxy. This course might also include examples of coding frameworks, coded data transcripts, or field memos.

2. **In-class mock exercises.** It is possible to give students some experience with data collection and analysis—however minimal—by incorporating small, targeted in-class exercises that allow for role-playing or simulated research activities. For example, we have had students conduct a truncated interview on a relatively benign issue in groups of three: one to interview, one to be interviewed, and one to observe the interaction. In such a scenario, you can provide prompts, allow for a brief preparation period, and then, after the task itself, hear

a debriefing from the three students both within their group and to the entire class.

3. **Low-stakes, real-world research simulations**. You might give your students a prompt for a more realistic data collection experience, usually outside of the classroom. This could entail student observation in a public space—interactions at a bus stop, for example. It could also involve student interviews with friends or family members (you can give an interview guide to the students or make guide development part of the assignment) about a general topic. Students might practice with a recorder; you might task them with taking field notes during or following the interview. We do caution, with these types of activities, that you pay special attention to the expectation of explicit and informed consent for those subject to the research gaze. While it's true that these activities are only practice research and not the real thing, you want to make sure you aren't modeling problematic practices in your course structures for first-time researchers.

4. **Analyze existing data**. Another project option would be to have students analyze publicly available data around a particular topic, such as documents, images, website content, and social media. While this approach would not have human interaction and therefore students would not be able to build skills around interviewing and social interactions, it can potentially supplement other discrete interviewing activities that occur in the classroom. For example, students could access and analyze sources of public health information and disinformation to understand effective health promotion campaigns. They could also be tasked with collecting and analyzing materials produced by various stakeholders with different perspectives and priorities, and with using the concepts of reflexivity and positionality to understand the contours of a particular debate in public health (e.g., e-cigarettes). One advantage of this approach is that it eliminates the need for IRB review given that the materials would be publicly available.

5. **Real research, with substantial support**. In our more advanced course series, we set up partnerships with local community-based organizations (CBOs), who work with us on a qualitative research project that a team of students can complete over time. Students meet with CBO representatives to understand their goals and priorities, develop a research plan, identify participants, collect data, analyze it, and present their findings to the CBO at the end of the course (Box 2.3). We find that our public health graduate students enjoy working on a real project, one where their findings will be of use to an organization. However, the timelines and logistical challenges of working with outside organizations—including engagement with IRB review by the course instructor as well as, potentially, by course students—mean this is a decision not to be made lightly. Such an approach also requires that instructors provide the student teams with substantial support to ensure that the work is both methodologically and ethically rigorous. While learning through structured and supported real-world experience can be the best way to master qualitative methods, this is also the most time-intensive approach for the instructor and the students. The necessary investments are such that there needs to be a clear justification for this approach.

Box 2.3 Tips and tricks: Class projects with Community-Based Organizations (CBOs)

Here are some of the strategies we've learned over many years of working with CBO partners on course projects:

- **Start planning early**. We suggest arranging student projects well *before* your course starts, then allowing students some latitude to decide which project they prefer.

continued

Box 2.3 *continued*

- **Set up times to meet with potential CBO partners** before your course starts and discuss their ideas for potential projects and goals for the collaboration. Why are they interested in partnering with the course—what are they looking to get out of any course project?

- **Make sure the CBOs know your course structure and expectations**. We create a handout of key points about the collaboration, including timelines (e.g., each student must complete their first interview by X date; final presentations will be held by Y date) and course project expectations (e.g., the number of interviews or focus groups each student will complete). In addition, the CBOs must understand *what you are asking of them*—Do they need to help identify potential participants? Recruit them? Schedule interviews?—and what the CBO will get in return: should they expect a final report? A presentation for their staff? Will they and/or participants be compensated?

- **Consider how much you are willing (and able) to adapt your course expectations and timelines** to the CBO's goals and ability to participate. You may decide to change the project in ways that work better for the CBO. For example, we typically expect students to conduct at least two forms of data collection (e.g., interviews and focus groups, or interviews and observation), but we have relaxed this expectation when CBOs could only offer the ability to conduct interviews. In other cases, you may decide that the CBO goals and course goals are too different for a collaboration to make sense. We declined projects after it became clear that the CBO really wanted a quantitative, survey-based approach, and a qualitative approach would not satisfy their needs.

- **Expect and prepare to positively respond to delays**. CBO timelines rarely align with course timelines. They are often short-staffed and busy, and your student project may not be a high priority for them even if they express interest and willingness to partner with course students. Plan for delays as much as possible and create alternative plans as needed. For example, during the course, we may tell students that if they are unable to connect with an interview participant by a given date, they can interview a classmate and turn that in for the assignment instead.

- **Consider the number of projects and the number of students per project**. Generally, we assign four to six students per CBO project. We find that, over the course of a semester, this number allows the whole team to collect data sufficient for meaningful answers to a CBO's research questions without leaving the team unwieldy.
- **Select one student team member to handle all communication with the CBO**. We find that CBOs find it challenging when several students send separate emails on different topics. Harmonizing team communication can help.
- As the faculty member, **connect with the CBO regularly to make sure that the project is going well, communication is clear, and expectations are being met.**
- **Consider using an end-of-project evaluation**, to be completed by both CBO collaborators and students. We have also used peer assessments, with team members assessing each other's contribution to group assignments to understand how individual students contributed to the team deliverables.
- **Decide how you might approach partnering with organizations multiple years in a row**. Some CBOs will want a one-time collaboration, others will be happy to collaborate each year, and still others will offer projects periodically or sporadically.

You can also adapt these suggestions to student team collaborations with other researchers, such as projects with faculty members or other groups. For example, slightly less intensive than a CBO project is to have students do on-campus projects or simulations as consultants. Students can work with recreation centers, student health centers, emergency management, or the office of sustainability on questions or act as pretend consultants to answer a generated research question of interest related to student health.

Class size

The number of students in a class impacts how those students will engage with you and with each other, as well as what you can assign. A seminar-style class with 15 or fewer students might incorporate in-depth discussions of assigned readings, written work with detailed instructor feedback, and in-class learning activities based on active participation and interaction among students. For larger classes, long-form written assignments may not be feasible due to the instructor's limited capacity to read and comment on every student's work. Because a larger class may also make it difficult for the instructor to keep every student engaged with and accountable for seminar-style reading discussions or case studies, these types of assignments might also be ill-advised. For such courses, we find it helpful to design brief, in-class exercises for students to work on in small groups, followed by a full-class debriefing.

Intensive courses

Sometimes we are called upon to teach qualitative methods over a compressed timeline, such as when training a field team, or as part of a specialized institute that develops the capacity of academics and researchers in other settings. Although students in an intensive course may receive the same number of contact hours they would in a more traditional course, an intensive course gives them less time to reflect, practice skills outside the classroom, and read background materials. Intensive courses can also be exhausting for both student and instructor. You might see this type of course as a precious opportunity to expose your students, who otherwise wouldn't have access to qualitative methods training, and be tempted to cover a lot of material. However, you should approach an intensive course with caution in relation to the amount of material that can be covered effectively. We have found that it is important to remain realistic about what the students can accomplish in a short period and how you can balance their exposure to ideas with the goal of mastering skills.

In general, we would recommend prioritizing using your time with students to interact rather than to communicate information. Based on our experience, here are several strategies to consider when preparing to teach an intensive course:

- **Consider either [a.] eliminating readings altogether or [b.] requiring students to prepare for the course by reading all of the necessary materials beforehand.** We do not recommend planning for students to read outside of class during the course period. We've had success assigning students preparatory videos or recorded lectures before the start of the course, as doing so allows us to spend more class time engaging with emergent issues or questions related to the didactic content.
- **Combine didactic content with applied and interactive components across the condensed timeline**. We recommend incorporating short exercises throughout the day.
- **Create opportunities for students to engage with each other and with the instructional team**. Interactions could include brief group activities, such as "Think-Pair-Share," a pedagogical technique where the instructor poses one or more open-ended questions and asks students to think quietly about them for a minute or two. Then each student pairs up with a partner and they discuss the question for up to five minutes. Finally, the whole class engages in group discussion about the most salient issues raised in the paired discussions. You can also put students into breakout groups to develop interview questions or discuss code definitions and have members of the instructional team visit each group.
- **Incorporate supports**—such as high levels of teaching assistant engagement—that allow students to get feedback on developing their ideas or applying concepts during the course.

Student considerations

To design an effective course, professors should consider their students and their needs in relation to their engagement with qualitative research coursework. Undergraduates, researchers, and practitioners will all have different backgrounds and training needs. Ideally, these needs will be reflected in specific course goals. As we outlined above, we develop our introductory courses to prepare a consumer of qualitative research to understand what qualitative methods are and how they can be useful. We have also developed and implemented courses that prepare students to understand qualitative methods, and to use them either as part of a research team or on their own fledgling project (usually a doctoral study). Often, our students are a mixture of these examples; regardless, it is essential that they understand what your course is intended to achieve.

The key directive regarding students' training is to **meet them where they are and take them where they need to go.** Students take a qualitative methods course for diverse reasons: some are public health practitioners who plan to incorporate qualitative approaches into their jobs; others do so to meet a requirement of their degree program or gain exposure to a wide range of methodological approaches. Still others have considerable hands-on experience and want to gain better foundational knowledge about the methods that they have already experienced. Students with different motivations are often seated next to each other in the same course. As an instructor, it is important that you make clear from the outset of each course what its goals are and what students can expect to learn upon completion, and how this will be accomplished.

Student background

A common challenge of teaching methods courses at the graduate level is the diversity of student expertise (Barraket, 2005). Just as it's important to consider students' motivations and goals for taking a class, it's also important to understand the exposure to qualitative approaches your students are likely to have when they come to class. For example, students with more of a background in social and behavioral sciences research might not need additional attention to generic issues pertaining to study design. At the same time, if students are steeped in principles and questions of a positivist, quantitative paradigm, the constructivist and interpretivist approach of qualitative research may be new and challenging for them. (For help with this situation, see Chapter 3, and our discussion of teaching theory.) In such a scenario, you are likely to need to dedicate some class time to getting everyone on the same page with the epistemological and theoretical paradigms that underpin qualitative approaches, broadening your students' understanding of what it means to conduct research and do science.

Student needs

It is our position that no qualitative methods course, however short, can afford to skip over the "whys" of qualitative research and go straight to the "hows," even if this is what students think that they need. Many students come to a qualitative course with the same few common questions, including the following:

- "How many people do I need to interview?" or "How many focus groups are enough?"
- "Who should moderate a focus group?"
- "Do you need consent to observe in a public place?"
- "Is it OK to ask different participants different questions in an in-depth interview?"

It is not enough, however, to design a course to simply provide factual answers to such questions. It is also critical to help your students understand *why* you answer these questions the way you do. Understanding the principles of qualitative research is crucial for good study design and will also help students respond to their colleagues' questions about the value and process of qualitative work, and provide a foundation for students' assessments of the rigor and quality of qualitative work they encounter throughout their careers.

You are likely to encounter many students who seek concrete skills, including how to manage qualitative data, how to conduct an interview, and how to work with qualitative data analysis software. Finding ways to offer these students an opportunity to build such skills is therefore a frequent priority in any course. When preparing for any course in which students will collect data, even just for practice, you will want to check with your institution's IRB for guidance on oversight requirements. It may be worthwhile to give your students opportunities to conduct mock interviews with classmates in lieu of or in addition to field assignments.

Special Considerations for Training Public Health Practitioners in Qualitative Research

Qualitative methods are a vital tool in public health practice, where practitioners apply these methods to program evaluation, community needs assessments, and policy development. In all our own courses—which often include a mix of academic researchers and public health practitioners—we incorporate foundational principles of qualitative methods (including epistemology), albeit to different degrees, depending on the specific learning objectives of the course. It is certainly the case that students working in applied settings may not need to explicitly reference foundational concepts in their work. We feel, however, that it is important to expose all students to the principles that explain why qualitative methods are conducted and analyzed the way that they are. Others may choose to not include epistemology as part of their courses that are intended to prepare students for applied research, but we have found that some consideration of the distinct approach to the nature of knowledge is appreciated by all students, including those who are seeking to be informed consumers of qualitative research rather than researchers themselves.

When training public health professionals in qualitative research, instructors should consider the following:

1. **Applied focus**. Unlike graduate students conducting research for dissertations, practitioners often need to apply qualitative methods in real-world settings with time and resource constraints. Emphasizing rapid assessment techniques, such as brief ethnographic interviews or focus groups, can be beneficial.

2. **Action-oriented analysis**. Public health practitioners typically use qualitative data to inform decision-making rather than to build theory. Training should emphasize practical frameworks such as thematic analysis for program improvement, rather than more abstract approaches like grounded theory.

3. **Interdisciplinary collaboration**. Public health work often involves collaboration across multiple disciplines, including epidemiology, social work, and policy studies. Practitioners may need guidance on how to integrate qualitative findings with quantitative data to create comprehensive public health insights.

4. **Ethical and cultural considerations**. Practitioners frequently engage with marginalized or vulnerable populations. Training should highlight ethical concerns such as informed consent, confidentiality in community settings, and the importance of culturally responsive research practices.

5. **Communication and stakeholder engagement**. Unlike academic researchers who primarily write for scholarly audiences, public health practitioners must often translate qualitative findings into actionable recommendations for policymakers, community leaders, and funding agencies. Teaching should include strategies for writing policy briefs and creating accessible reports.

Faculty considerations

Reflexivity is an important concept to cover in a qualitative course—and it is likewise important that instructors of qualitative methods courses in public health engage in reflexive practice with their own teaching. As you plan, deliver, and evaluate your course, ask yourself the following questions:

- Who are you as a teacher, and how does this relate to what this course is intended to achieve?
- What are your own goals for teaching this course?
- How do you relate to your students?
- How are aspects of your identity likely to shape what your students take from the course?
- How does this course fit within your life and professional practice?

There is no perfect combination of answers to these questions. Thinking about them and about their influence on how you implement your course and how your students receive it is, however, a worthwhile activity.

Resources

As a faculty member, your resources and support for teaching will vary depending on—among other things—your institution; whether there are other qualitative researchers in your program, department, or school; any ongoing research projects in which students can participate; whether you can call upon a center dedicated to pedagogical issues; and the existence of collaborations with community organizations on which students can work. Assessing the available resources and how to incorporate them into your course can help create a more immersive class, one that presents qualitative methods as your students might encounter them outside the classroom.

Teaching style

Many of the teaching strategies we recommend in this book and practice in our own classes involve a lot of hands-on learning and discussion and less emphasis on lectures and information dissemination modalities. When designing your class, consider the extent to which you are comfortable moving away from lectures and sharing more control of how each class unfolds with your students, or flipping your classroom so that students complete the course's didactic aspects on their own and use their time together for experiential learning.

Team teaching

We teach many of our qualitative classes as a two-, three-, or even four-faculty team. You might seek an opportunity to teach as part of a team, or the decision may be made for you by whomever in your department assigns course responsibilities. Whatever the circumstance, keep in mind that team teaching can have many strengths. It can allow for a division of labor, making the course easier to complete. This also might make it possible for each team member to take responsibility for the class elements in which they have specific expertise or interest—a faculty member who regularly uses observation in their own work may be better prepared to cover that topic than one who relies primarily on interviews. If one member of your teaching team uses different approaches to qualitative analysis in their own work, your students may benefit from seeing that instructor's perspective. In our own team-taught courses, we feel that our students benefit from seeing a variety of qualitative studies throughout the class: both international and domestic, policy-oriented and more evaluation-oriented, and which address a mulitple public health topics.

However, team teaching also poses potential challenges. To avoid a disjointed class, one in which students must contend with contradictory messages, overlapping content, or gaps, it is vital that faculty members know what their colleagues are teaching and how they teach it. If time allows, and particularly in your first year team-teaching a course, we suggest that faculty members sit in on each other's classes. This benefits every group member's instruction by facilitating a collegial atmosphere in the classroom, one in which the observing faculty member might chime in here and there to add comments and examples, and reference ideas slated for later class sessions.

Instructor background and experience

As you populate your course syllabus and plan lessons, we encourage you to keep with qualitative principles and call upon your own experiences conducting qualitative research—from your most-seasoned and exemplary to your most cringeworthy. Speaking sincerely about what you've seen and done in the field and the lessons you've learned from your actions can make for engaging and powerful learning opportunities. In our own sample interview guides and codebooks, we often reference our most recent work—as well as that from our own student days. We share what we liked about these tools and how they served our analysis, and talk about what we would do differently if we had the opportunity. This kind of presentation can begin as didactic and then evolve into a group discussion. Such an approach can break the mystique that research (and researchers!) must be perfect and encourage routine reflection and learning. It can also give students the space to imagine their own processes and engage in realistic decision-making. Additionally, we like to share any articles and books we're reading to make it clear that we, too, are still learning—and to further challenge the idea of an unbreachable divide between student and teacher. We are all hopefully methodological learners for as long as we undertake research.

Colleagues and collaborators

It can be very powerful for students to hear more experienced researchers (who could, depending on the context, still be relative novices themselves) discuss their experiences. To us, this isn't a didactic process as much as it's another reflexive practice. Just as we learn in qualitative research from giving people a chance to talk to us in their own words, so too can it be powerful to have people share or answer open-ended questions about their own research experiences. Do you have colleagues with whom you can collaborate? If so, can you bring them into the classroom to talk about what they do, how they do it, and what they've learned in the process? Such guest speakers don't necessarily need to be experts in qualitative methods; in fact, your students may learn more from someone just a little further along than they are and who likely dealt with issues similar to the ones they can expect to encounter in the field. But that's also not to discount a special guest with a great deal of experience, who might be very well equipped to reflect upon why things went well in one instance and poorly in another.

You might ask any colleagues to talk about one or more of the following:

- What was the most recent qualitative data collection approach you used? Why did you choose that approach?
- How do you prepare for a qualitative interview?
- Give us an example of an interview that went surprisingly well or surprisingly poorly. In hindsight, do you know why it turned out the way it did?
- Do you have any tips for doing your first observation?
- What are some of your strategies for gaining access to an observational setting?
- How do you keep people on topic during an interview?
- Are there groups of people or topics you think don't work well as a focus group?
- How do you take field notes, and how do you use them?

Remember, though, that you aren't off the hook for the class just because someone else is in front of the class. Speakers still must be managed—you must decide how they fit into your syllabus and which learning objectives you want to address with each guest lecture. If you plan to assess students based on these sessions, you need to make sure that the message of each lecture is in harmony with your syllabus. We also suggest being present for guests whenever possible. While it can be useful to invite guests for days when a conflict will keep you out of the classroom (and is sometimes necessary to do so), if you're present, you'll be better able to understand how their lecture fits with the rest of your course, ensure the guest's messages are consistent (or react if they are not), and interact with the speaker in ways that show your students how the material connects to things they've already been taught.

Including data management in your course

In any course where the goal is preparing students to collect their own data, it's a good idea to include material on data management. Data management is often overlooked as a skill—but it is hugely important for effective research. Learning good data management skills and best practices and thinking about data management from the beginning of a research project can lead to more rigorous and higher quality studies. Qualitative research can generate a lot of data and a lot of different *types* of data—interview transcripts, interview recordings, reflexivity notes, memos, field notes, documents, coded data, and even short quantitative surveys! Good data management throughout the life of a project minimizes the chance of any single piece of data going missing and undermining the integrity of the project.

Consider one example of how critical a careful approach to data management can be. Assume that a student's analytic goal is to understand the differences in how two populations think about or experience a public health problem. To meet their goal, this student will need to be able to document characteristics of the different populations systematically so they can conduct subgroup analyses later. The student will also need to establish methods for eliciting and recording this information. Good data management practices will enable the student to address each of these issues (see Box 2.4 for an example of a data management activity).

Box 2.4 Tips and tricks: Data management activity overview

In this activity, students will engage in a practical exercise where they are tasked with organizing and managing a hypothetical qualitative research project's data. Through this exercise, they will experience firsthand the challenges and best practices in qualitative data management.

Materials needed:

- **case study**: a brief description of a hypothetical qualitative research project (interviews, field notes, audio recordings, etc.)
- **data samples**: mock qualitative data (transcripts, audio recordings, photos, field notes)
- **data management tools**: printed templates for data organization (folders, labels, index cards)
- **access to computers** (optional for electronic storage simulation)
- **checklist for data management best practices** (provided by the instructor)

Instructions:

1. **Introduction** (10 minutes):
   a. Begin by explaining the significance of good data management in qualitative research. Highlight the following key points:
      i. data integrity: ensures that data is accurate, complete, and can be reliably referenced

continued

Box 2.4 *continued*

---

    ii. accessibility: helps researchers access data easily and quickly when needed

    iii. security: protects sensitive data from unauthorized access

    iv. ethical considerations: ensures confidentiality and informed consent

    v. long-term storage and retrieval: supports the future usability of the data.

2. **Assign groups** (five minutes):

    a. Divide students into small groups (three to four students per group).

    b. Each group will be given a **Case Study** involving a qualitative research project and **Data Samples** (e.g., interview transcripts, field notes, audio recordings).

    c. The case study should describe the type of qualitative research (e.g., interviews, ethnography, focus groups) and the data collected, including sensitive or private information that requires ethical handling.

3. **Data organization challenge** (20 minutes):

    a. Each group's task is to organize the data based on best practices for qualitative data management:

        i. **Step 1: Categorize and label**: Groups will categorize different data (transcripts, notes, audio files, etc.), label them clearly, and create a simple organization system (e.g., using folders, binders, or virtual files if using a computer).

        ii. **Step 2: Document the metadata**: Each group will fill out a metadata template that includes important information such as the source of the data, date of collection, any ethical considerations (e.g., anonymization), and relevant context.

        iii. **Step 3: Plan for storage and security**: Students will discuss how they would store and secure the data, considering physical storage (e.g., locked cabinets) or digital storage (e.g., password-protected files, encrypted cloud storage).

   iv. **Step 4: Ethical considerations**: Students should consider how to anonymize data or handle sensitive information, ensuring the privacy and confidentiality of research participants.

4. **Group presentations** (15 minutes):
   a. After organizing the data, each group will present their data management strategy to the class.
   b. They will explain:
      i. how they organized the data (methods/tools used)
      ii. how they ensured the data was secure and ethically handled
      iii. any challenges they faced in managing the data.

5. **Class discussion** (10 minutes):
   a. After all groups have presented, facilitate a class discussion on the key takeaways:
      i. What went well in their data management strategies?
      ii. What were some potential risks or issues they identified during the exercise?
      iii. How can poor data management affect the quality and credibility of qualitative research?
   b. Provide real-world examples of data breaches or ethical violations in research to illustrate the importance of good data management.

Wrap-up and reflection (5 minutes):

- Ask students to reflect individually on the importance of data management in qualitative research by writing a brief response to the following prompts:
   o Why is good data management crucial for maintaining the credibility of qualitative research?

What specific strategies or tools do you plan to use in your own research to manage your data effectively?

Packing for the classroom like you pack for the field

As researchers and educators, we notice many similarities when our activities go well and when they don't. One important contributing factor is thought and preparation well ahead of time. This means treating our classroom prep almost identically to what we do when preparing for the field (Figure 2.2). Below is a list of items we suggest you consider putting in your teaching suitcase, and whether you think you'll need them on a given educational journey.

- sample interview and focus group guides
- sample consent forms
- research plans
- observational guides/recording sheets
- data sets (coded and uncoded)
- data excerpts
- grading rubrics
- teaching/demo licenses to software programs for analysis
- recorded lectures
- guest colleagues and guidance for them
- IRB agreements for field or practice activities
- partnerships with community organizations

Summary

In our experience, teaching qualitative methods and practicing them in the field are very similar in that they each require you to prepare as best you can and be ready to adapt as you go. Some things will go as planned (and maybe even better!); others may not go anywhere near how you thought that they would. But it's perfectly fine to make modifications along the way, based on what you're learning. It's our hope and expectation that, by the end of every course, we have learned important lessons along with our students. In that spirit, try to revisit

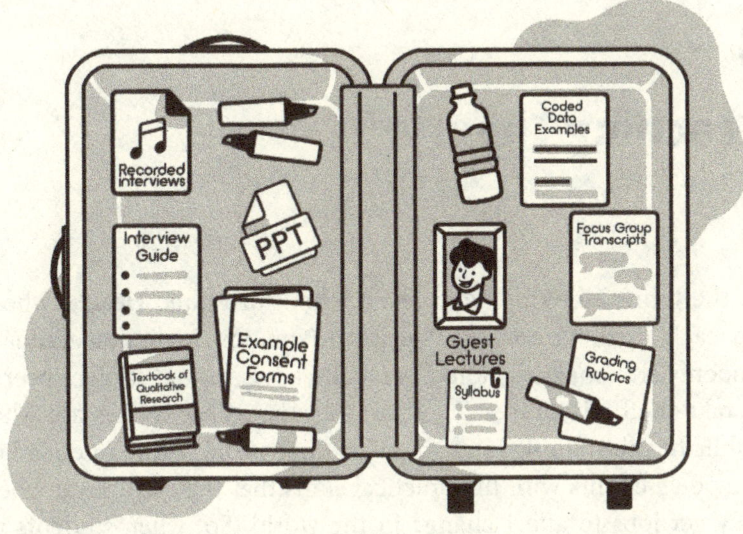

Figure 2.2 Packing for the classroom

your learning objectives regularly as the course progresses. Ask yourself if what you've been doing and what you have planned will get you to those objectives. If the answer is no, how can you pivot so that you meet your students where they are (and yourself where it turns out you are) and refocus yourself to successfully proceed on an altered path to the same destination?

3

Teaching Theory

At the Johns Hopkins Bloomberg School of Public Health, where we teach, methods are king. During orientation, incoming graduate students are repeatedly told (by faculty advisors and student peers) to take methods classes. They are told that these classes are what public health training is all about; methods courses are intended to provide students with the practical skills that they will need when they get jobs to affect change in the world. So, when students in our school enroll in a qualitative research class, they expect practical methods training. They want to learn the tools of the trade: how to conduct in-depth interviews, how to facilitate focus groups, and perhaps also how to undertake participant observation and analyze documents. We are firm believers that doing this work well is critical, and we have devoted Chapter 5 of this book to training students in these methods. We don't believe, however, that a good qualitative methods class can focus solely on practical skills. Theory is also critically important, and a thoughtful use of theory often allows for the strongest insights from qualitative studies (Figure 3.1).

Can you teach methods without teaching theory?

Theory is regularly considered to be about thinking instead of doing, and to therefore be the opposite of practice. Students may wonder what the point is of learning about theory in an applied field like public health. After all, do you need to know theory to be a good public health researcher? Well, we argue that, yes—you very much

Teaching Qualitative Research in Public Health. Katherine Clegg Smith et al., Oxford University Press.
© Oxford University Press (2026). DOI: 10.1093/9780197662472.003.0003

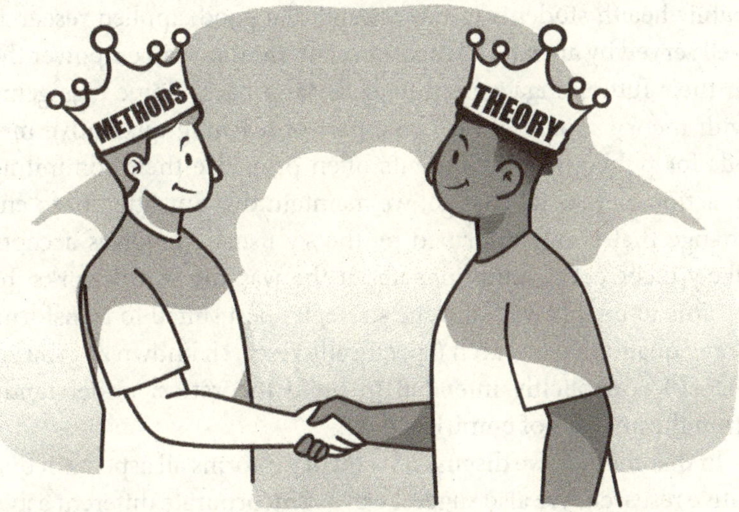

Figure 3.1 Methods and theory are both critically important for rigorous and impactful qualitative research

do! Without understanding epistemology, theoretical perspective, and methodology:

- How can a researcher select which methods to use?
- How will they know which concepts to explore?
- How will they interpret their findings?

But while theory is critical for a quality research endeavor, and even understanding a quality research endeavor, figuring out how to connect engagement and explanatory ideas in a methods class where students want to learn how to do public health research can be a tricky dance indeed.

We believe theory is an essential underpinning of good qualitative practice and good public health—you cannot do one without the other. Kawulich (2016) has asserted, "Theory, both tacit and explicit, is an integral part of the research process from beginning to end" (p. 47). Theories inform the questions we ask and our exploration of how phenomena relate to each other. Encouraging public health students to understand that good, applied research is well served by an explicit theoretical orientation can empower them in their future engagement with the approach. Some engagement with theory should always be a part of teaching qualitative methods for public health. Students often prioritize their commitment to action and social change; we maintain that any attempt to enact change that is not informed by theory usually involves accepting likely incorrect assumptions about the way the world works, how it came to be this way, and the strategies best suited to transform it. Some qualitative research (specifically research known as grounded theory) is explicitly intended to build theoretical understanding from the analysis of empirical data.

In this chapter, we discuss how theory informs all aspects of qualitative research. We also suggest ways to incorporate different aspects of theory into your qualitative classes.

Epistemology: How we understand the world

In each of our courses, whenever we talk about theory, we begin with **epistemology**. The concept refers not to a specific theory to be built or tested in a research project, but rather to fundamental assumptions about the nature of knowledge. Epistemology is part of the philosophy of science and of the larger paradigm in which we conduct research.

Epistemological questions include:

- How can we learn about the world?
- What kinds of knowledge are possible or legitimate?
- What do we think we are doing when we are doing research?
- How do we know things?
- What are the sources of our knowledge?
- What does it mean to say we know something?
- How do we justify what we believe or know?

In our courses, we introduce three epistemological approaches: **objectivism**, **constructivism**, and **subjectivism**. Because these ideas and comparisons are generally new for students, we find that it is important to make space and opportunities for active engagement with them.

- **Objectivism** posits that there is an external reality, that this reality can be known, and that truth resides in the object of research, independent of the researcher. From an objectivist perspective, the goal of research is to reduce bias and find the sole existing truth.
- **Constructivism**, by contrast, argues that there is no single, objective reality.— The goal of research is the understanding of reality from relevant perspectives while accounting for the influence of the researcher and the research interaction on the knowledge generated. Research is cocreated through the interaction between the researcher and the person or object being studied.
- **Subjectivism** contends that meaning is **not** the result of an interplay between the researcher and the object of research. Rather, meaning is imposed by the researcher on their object. Thus, there is no reality independent of the research enterprise: the action of research creates infinite realities. (We also note that few—if any—public health researchers are subjectivists. We primarily introduce this concept as something of a boundary to help students better understand constructivism.)

It can be challenging to get students to understand the differences between these epistemological perspectives. It is, however, a critical foundation for understanding qualitative methods. We find it helpful to provide familiar analogies and prompts—such as Patton's baseball analogy (see Box 3.1 and Figure 3.2)—as students work through the three distinct stances. In addition, we typically include a class exercise (Box 3.2 and Figure 3.3) in which we show our students a photograph of either a tree or a cow, then ask them to apply each of the three epistemological perspectives to answer this question: What is that? You could also use the example of maps to compare different epistemological approaches (Box 3.3).

Box 3.1 Tips and tricks: Using a baseball analogy to introduce epistemology

We find many U.S. students can relate to the following example from Patton (2002) to help them understand the different epistemological perspectives.

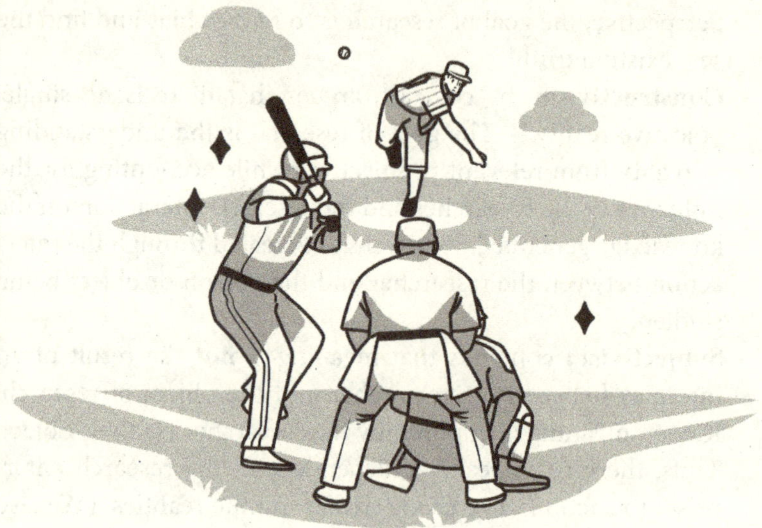

Figure 3.2 A baseball analogy to illustrate different epistemologies

Baseball umpires on the difference between a ball and a strike:

- Objectivist: "I call them as they are."
- Constructivist: "I call them as I see them."
- Subjectivist: "They ain't nothing until I call them."

Researchers on different understandings of "truth":

- Objectivist: "I can show you truth revealed by the data."
- Constructivist: "I can show you multiple truths held concurrently."
- Subjectivist: "Truth depends on one's consciousness."

Box 3.2 Tips and tricks: Class exercise contrasting epistemological approaches to everyday objects

One of the ways in which we engage students in epistemology is to show the class a photo of an "everyday" object and ask students to name it. Then, we prompt them to consider it from the three different episte-mological perspectives. It can work well to model this for one or two objects and then engage the students for another one or more additional objects.

Objectivist: That is an animal. That is a mammal. That is a cow.

Constructivist: Yes—that is an animal, mammal, and cow. It can also be seen as a source of income. It is also a source of pollution. People with certain religious backgrounds see it as a sacred animal. The mean-ing of this object is determined by your perspective and your engagement with it.

Subjectivist: That is pretty. That is art. Calling it a pig is as valid a perspec-tive as any other.

Objectivist: That is a tree.

Constructivist: An arborist will see something very different in this photo than most people. They may identify the species of tree or notice some-thing specific about it—that it is growing in a certain way or that it is diseased. Someone whose parents are buried under this tree may see something else in the photo. The photo's meaning is partly determined by their perspective, as well as by the patterns on the page.

Subjectivist: Each interpretation of this photo is equally valid. The arborist who sees a specific species of tree is no more correct than the person who calls this a photo of the modern condition. Meaning does not come from an interaction between the photo and the viewer; the viewer imposes meaning upon the photo.

Objectivist: That is a blood pressure cuff that can tell someone if they have high blood pressure. Blood pressure can be measured accurately. High blood pressure indicates a health problem, or at least the risk of one.

continued

Box 3.2 *continued*

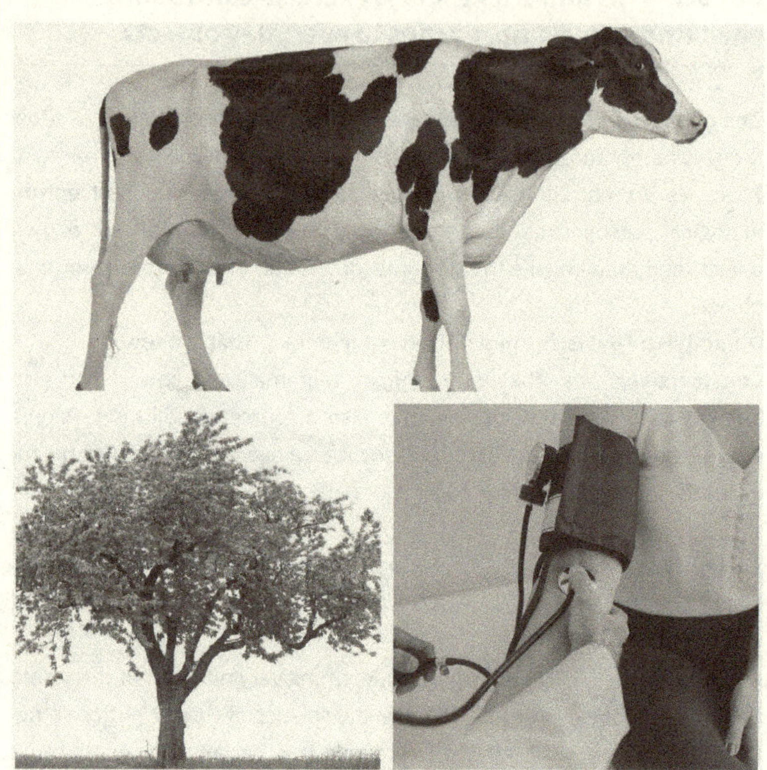

Figure 3.3   A cow, tree, and blood pressure cuff as prompts for class discussions of epistemology (iStock.com/GlobalP (Cow), iStock.com/Sieboldianus (tree), iStock.com/andreswd (blood pressure cuff))

Constructivist: Blood pressure is measured using a blood pressure cuff. Many variables can affect their measurements, including the ability of the person using the cuff and the context in which they use it. The blood pressure level considered normal has changed over time, reflecting changing scientific understandings, social structures, and expectations.

Subjectivist: Blood pressure is a social construct. Society has chosen to create the concept of blood pressure and to measure it in a certain way;

the idea of blood pressure would not exist if it had not been named by people and thus created as a concept. Other ways of understanding whether someone is at risk of a stroke, such as observing them, could be equally legitimate.

Box 3.3 Tips and tricks: Class exercise contrasting epistemological approaches using maps

You can also use maps to explore epistemology. Like research, maps are a representation of the world. Present several different maps of your local city or area. An objectivist might say that a map is a depiction of a place—it tells you what is in the place and how the elements of the place relate to one another spatially, and there are maps that correctly or incorrectly represent that space. However, a constructivist would see a map as a historical and social product. It depicts a particular view of what is important to know about a place and reflects the social organization at the time of its creation—a map of hiking trails in your city would be different from a map of queer-friendly spaces, and both would differ from a street map or a topographical map. Finally, a subjectivist would see that maps are products of specific people or groups in power, and they may bear little resemblance to any "truth" outside of those creating and using them for specific purposes.

In relation to these exercises, we spend the most time contrasting the objectivist and constructivist perspectives, as we feel this comparison is the most relevant one for public health researchers. We emphasize how epistemology influences our thinking about both the overall goals of research and the specific elements, like reflexivity and rigor, of how we come to understand whether research has been done well. We note that most qualitative researchers identify with a constructivist perspective and encourage our students to reflect on the researcher's role in producing knowledge. It has been our experience that students at all levels engage in these exercises.

On several occasions, we have had physician or lab science students who are taking our courses with a goal of understanding qualitative methods tell us that these exercises were highly valuable not only for their understanding of qualitative methods, but for science overall.

In more advanced classes, we discuss epistemology in greater depth, exploring its relationship to several aspects of research, including:

- **The process of knowing**: Objectivism is concerned with bias and replicability; constructivism is concerned with positionality and reflexivity.
- **The products of research**: Objectivism focuses on producing objective scientific knowledge, accurate and certain because it is discovered, not created; constructivism's interpretations are always anchored in a particular historical, political, and social context.
- **Research design**: Objectivist studies are designed to ensure minimal bias; constructivist studies are open-ended and iterative to allow for perspectives to be generated.
- **The processes of analysis and writing**: Objectivism's goal is the discovery of a single true story; constructivism is engaged with presenting multiple stories.
- **Diverse perspectives**: Constructivism is enriched and expanded through Indigenous and other cross-cultural and diverse ways of knowing. An advanced class might read Linda Tuhiwai Smith's (2013) book *Decolonizing Methodologies: Research and Indigenous Peoples* and incorporate its lessons into classroom discussions and exercises, and course assignments.

We cover these topics because we feel it's important for students to grasp not just *what* epistemology is, but *how* it influences the very tangible, practical elements of a qualitative study. An objectivist approach will yield a different process and final product than a constructivist approach; advanced students should be able to articulate how a given epistemological approach relates to specific methodological decisions. In Box 3.4, we discuss other activities and ways of engaging your students in discussions about different epistemological approaches.

Box 3.4 Qualitative building blocks: Isn't all this just fake news?

We live in a highly polarized news environment, and there has been a considerable democratization of knowledge with the advance of social media. Given this context, we have noted that students now often ask a question about constructivist and subjectivist epistemologies along the lines of: "Are these epistemological approaches just 'alternative facts' or 'fake news'?"

From a subjectivist perspective, perhaps all facts can be fake. Subjectivists argue that we make sense of our world by imposing meaning onto it; meaning does not exist until the researcher creates it. By this logic, any meaning imposed on the world could be valid, and any fact could be considered fake.

But this is not the case from a constructivist perspective. The constructivist will tell you that you can't come to any interpretation you want based on what you observe or study. Acknowledging that the researcher shapes the products of their research does not make all interpretations equally valid. Meanings are constructed in a social context: an interpretation is invalid if it is without utility for others who share the same context. For the constructivist, it is quite possible for one's interpretation to be incorrect.

We give the analogy of a journalist whose job is to describe world events that are inherently complex. The journalist must boil down that complexity into a 500-word article by making all kinds of decisions about which facts to include, how to frame the story in relation to previous events, and what other information they need to help the reader understand why an event is newsworthy. Their job is to interact with the truth and try to represent it as faithfully as possible. Different journalists writing about the same event will produce different articles unique in their own ways, even if working

continued

Box 3.4 *continued*

---

with the same set of parameters (including word length, outlet, timeframe, and audience). But that doesn't mean that they can write whatever they want. They still need to be attentive to facts as they discover and learn about them, and to represent, from their point of view, the elements of the story as faithfully and understandably as they can.

In the same way, constructivists acknowledge that their identities, experiences, and beliefs will shape the way that they think about the world. Because research requires interacting with the world as they find it and being true to what they hear from and observe about participants, it is through the process of interaction—or cocreation—that research is produced.

Theory does not, however, totally determine method. Crotty (1998) argued that "the distinction between qualitative and quantitative research occurs at the level of methods. It does not occur at the level of epistemology or theoretical perspective" (p. 14). In other words, qualitative research that uses interviews can be conducted from either a constructivist or an objectivist epistemological perspective. However, it's easier to align some epistemological stances, theoretical perspectives, methodologies, and methods than others. For example, symbolic interactionism (Blumer, 2013) as a theoretical perspective may fit easiest with a constructivist epistemology and with in-depth interviews as a method. On the other hand, if you were to use social cognitive theory (Bandura, 1986) to explore a behavior, you might be inclined to adopt an objectivist epistemology and use close-ended surveys to construct Likert scale responses as a method of inquiry.

We think it fair to say that most current qualitative researchers in public health identify as constructivists. Historically, most *quantitative* research was (and may still be) conducted from an objectivist perspective. But we've had many great class discussions about how a constructivist epistemology can and should apply to quantitative research. If you give your students the space to think about epistemology, you'll see them start to realize that survey questions do not necessarily tap into some mysterious truth that is waiting to be uncovered—survey data can also be understood as coconstructed knowledge shaped as much by the researcher who worded the questions and response options as by the participant's experience or the attitude they reflected in their answer choices. This understanding can, in turn, lend itself to a class debate, with one side arguing that survey research findings are by their nature coconstructed (or constructivist) and another that, if the researcher is careful in removing bias, their findings can reflect reality free of their influence (i.e., objectivist).

Alternatively, you might ask students to do a "Think-Pair-Share" exercise, in which they consider and then discuss with a partner whether they believe all research should be undertaken from a particular epistemological perspective or whether different types of research can be approached legitimately from different theoretical perspectives. We've been pleased to note that many of our students find their understanding of all types of public health research—not just qualitative—expanded by epistemological discussions like these.

When in a qualitative methods course should you teach theory?

Wagner et al. (2019) have raised the issue of when a qualitative course should address theory. Epistemological considerations and the philosophy of science are essential components of research training, but should you first whet your students' interest through experiential engagement with one or more of the data collection methods? After all, this is what many students will expect from a methods course.

Because we find it hard to talk about concepts like reflexivity and rigor without tying them to epistemology, we prefer to introduce epistemology and theoretical perspectives at the start of a course, framing them as the foundations upon which students can then build their understanding of methods. We return to this foundation throughout the course to demonstrate how our students' epistemological and theoretical perspectives will inform many of their practical decisions throughout the qualitative research process, including conceptualizing research questions, selecting appropriate methods, asking interview questions, and analyzing data.

Different conceptualizations of theory

With in-depth or advanced courses, you may want to help students think about the different ways in which the concept of theory is used. Crotty (1998) provided a framework that we find helpful for breaking down what theory is and how it fits into a researcher's general understanding of the research process. Crotty outlined a process of scaffolded learning in which students take concepts they may have learned in other classes, such as social cognitive theory, structure-functionalism, or stigma, and see how they align with epistemology and methods as part of an overall qualitative project. This application makes the overarching idea of theory more concrete and allows students to see how different aspects of theory can influence a qualitative study's design. In so doing, it can also help students design a coherent study, justify the choices they make, and help them interpret qualitative literature.

Crotty (1998, p. 3) identified four elements of the research process:

- **Epistemology**: "The theory of knowledge embedded in the theoretical perspective and thereby in the methodology"—e.g., objectivism, constructivism, and subjectivism, as discussed above.
- **Theoretical perspective**: "The philosophical stance informing the methodology and thus providing a context for the process and grounding its logic and criteria." As we explain later, such stances include symbolic interactionism, critical inquiry, feminism, or postmodernism.
- **Methodology**: "The strategy, plan of action, process, or design lying behind the choice and use of particular methods and linking the choice and use of methods to desired outcomes."

Methodologies, which we will cover in Chapter 4, can include ethnography, phenomenology, grounded theory, and action research.

- **Methods**: "The techniques or procedures used to gather and analyze data related to some research question or hypothesis." Some examples of methods are interviews, focus groups, and observation; we cover methods in greater depth in Chapter 5.

Crotty also described how these elements come together to shape a research study. For example, a study that uses critical race theory (theoretical perspective) and is grounded in constructivism (epistemology) could take an ethnographic approach (methodology) through participant observation and interviews (methods). You might have your students work out how each element applies to their own research projects or to selected published articles. Crotty also emphasized that some choices fit better than others because they contain complementary assumptions about the way the world works. In Box 3.5, we present a class exercise on matching epistemology, theoretical perspective, methodology, and methods in a way that "flows."

Box 3.5 Tips and tricks: Class exercise on matching epistemology, theoretical perspective, methodology, and methods

---

In courses where the goal is to build competence in study design (particularly for doctoral students), once your students are familiar with the concepts of epistemology, theoretical perspective, methodology, and methods, you can try this class exercise. Explain that some aspects of theory contain complementary assumptions about the way the world works. Other assumptions, though, may clash, creating tensions or inconsistencies if used as part of the same project. For example, critical race theory and constructivist epistemology both assume that social perceptions shape

continued

> **Box 3.5** *continued*
>
> ---
>
> reality; however, these might feel at odds with an objectivist epistemology. In your class exercise, provide a concrete example for each category and ask whether they fit together. For example, does a constructivist epistemology fit with critical inquiry as a theoretical perspective and case study as a methodology? Yes! Does an objectivist epistemology fit with queer theory as a theoretical perspective and ethnography as a methodology? Maybe the latter two work together, but they might not flow well with an objectivist epistemology.

Theory as a guide for analytical questions

In our introductory courses, we emphasize epistemology. In courses with more advanced students, we also cover theoretical perspectives and methodologies. In such courses, we are looking to engage students in nuanced discussions of how they might use theory in qualitative research, differentiating between applicable theories, conceptual models, and theorizing data. It is important to remember that everyone makes theoretical assumptions going into a study, whether or not they recognize this and state their assumptions in their dissemination of findings. When we do make our assumptions clear and can justify our choices—that's when the best research happens. We encourage our students to identify their theoretical orientations, what influences their questions, and how they interpret data to help them join an intellectual community with their use of theory.

Crotty (1998) has described theoretical perspectives as the philosophical stances that build on assumptions about how the world works and therefore provide context for one's research process. Examples of theoretical perspectives include queer theory, critical race theory, feminism, structural functionalism, and conflict theory. Most theoretical perspectives can be applied to many research topics and offer ideas or concepts—as well as the relationships between those concepts—that can shape research questions.

Theoretical perspectives exist on two levels of abstraction: **substantive theory** and **formal theory**. **Substantive theory** is developed for a specific area of social concern: understanding a social phenomenon like a street gang, for example, or a strike action, community cohesion, divorce, or race relations. A substantive theory is considered transferable, rather than generalizable, in the sense that while its elements develop relative to one set of circumstances, its context may be applicable to other entities or circumstances with similar characteristics. In contrast, **formal theories** can be applied to a wider context and may be built by considering findings or substantive theories from multiple studies. Formal theories are akin to what Timmermans and Tavory (2022) have called "grammatical theories": they were developed for a broad conceptual area in general theory, such as deviance, socialization, or power. Box 3.6 lists some examples of substantive and formal theories.

Box 3.6 Qualitative building blocks: Examples of substantive and formal theories for the classroom

Substantive theories

- stigma mechanisms among people living with HIV
- framing of the impact of climate change on health in the U.S. news media
- self-efficacy for dietary change
- development of a particular health care or social welfare system
- how women who use drugs negotiate their identities as mothers
- the relationship between family context and understanding genetic risk

Formal theories

- Social Cognitive Theory (Bandura, 1986)
- Implementation Theory (Proctor et al., 2011)

continued

> **Box 3.6** *continued*
>
> ---
>
> - Fundamental Causes of Disease (Link & Phelan, 1995)
> - Biopower and discipline (Foucault, 1998)
> - Bureaucratic Rationality (Weber; in Gerth et al., 2013)
> - Structural Violence (Farmer et al., 2016)
> - Intersectionality (Crenshaw, 1989; Bowleg, 2008)
> - Theory of Gender and Power (Connell, 2013)
> - Medicalization (Conrad, 1992)

Advanced students (and doctoral students in particular) may wonder how these discussions of theory fit with the **conceptual frameworks** they are often expected to develop as part of their dissertation proposals. We explain that a conceptual framework is an application of theory as it relates to a particular study or topic: it may use terms or constructs from a theoretical perspective and will demonstrate specific relationships among these constructs.

As a class exercise or a homework assignment, you could have students apply a specific theoretical perspective to an example research problem and see how it shapes the questions a study might ask and the methods they might choose to answer them. You could begin with the Health Belief Model (HBM), developed in the 1950s by social psychologists working for the U.S. Public Health Service (Rosenstock, 1974). The HBM proposes a set of individual-level constructs, among them the perceived severity of a given disease or health issue, perceived susceptibility to that disease or health issue, and cues to action, which are assumed to influence an individual's health-related behaviors. The HBM case would align with qualitative questions about how individuals perceive the issue and how susceptible they feel they are to this disease. In analysis, the researcher might create coding categories a priori from HBM constructs, scouring the data for examples of cues to action or perceived susceptibility. The example's theoretical perspective shapes multiple aspects of the study design, conduct, and analysis.

While we believe that students should engage with multiple substantive and formal theoretical perspectives in thinking about the application of qualitative methods, it is also important to acknowledge that qualitative inquiry may have different goals than the testing of theory. Some qualitative studies may be very descriptive, seeking to answer a question that is really as basic as "What is going on here?" and relying heavily on an emic perspective gathered through in-depth interviews. Theory is useful for going beyond a purely descriptive inquiry and asking questions such as, "*Why* is this happening?" or "*How* does this work?" Answering "why" and "how" questions requires us to engage with theory either explicitly or implicitly. Asking analytic questions about the data to understand a field's essential features (e.g., study site, population) and relationships among them will require engagement with substantive theories. And to understand what it all means and interpret the findings you may well have to engage with more formal theories. As Timmermans and Tavory (2022, p. 31) have reminded us, theory allows you to strengthen your argument and see surprises in your data. Beyond that, it's a way to connect your fieldwork to a larger scholarly conversation and expand the reach of your work.

One frame to help students link data to formal theory is Alasuutair's (1996) hourglass model. In this approach, the qualitative research process is a case analysis of a bounded system, contextualized within a larger historical and cultural framework. Rather than an attempt to formulate a universal grand theory, the task is the use of theory to illuminate a historical moment through the case being analyzed.

- Start with the broad theoretical/structural framework.
- Place the particular research site/population in this larger context and validate the choice of the specific case study.
- As research is the epicenter of the hourglass, analyze, in detail, a specific, closely defined object of study as a world of its own.
- Assess and discuss your results within the broader framework.

The hourglass model suggests that we often begin by generating substantive theory from data and then letting formal theory, or revisions to existing formal theory, emerge from substantive theory, rather than deducing substantive theory from formal theory. As studies generate and refine substantive theory, they will also feed into the process of generating and improving formal theory.

Box 3.7 provides additional ideas for how to incorporate theory, based on examples from our own courses.

Box 3.7 Tips and tricks: Teaching theory

We sometimes struggle with ways to incorporate theory—whether epistemology, specific theoretical or conceptual frameworks, or grand ideas about the way societies work—into our own courses. As we noted in Chapter 2, there are many factors to consider regarding the integration of theory into methods courses, among them the diversity of students' exposure to theory, motivations for taking the class, and the available time.

As you might expect, we have found some ways to be more successful than others. In one advanced qualitative data analysis course, we used to have students read theoretically grounded articles and book-length texts that complemented the course data set. While this approach did lead to interesting discussions and analytic insights into the data, in the end, our students simply did not have the time or headspace to fully grapple with the texts' theoretical concepts. As a result, we have moved away from assigning extensive texts, even in advanced courses. In later iterations of the course, we instead used Timmermans and Tavory's (2022) work on abductive analysis, which emphasizes the interplay between data and theory but does not teach any specific theoretical perspective.

In the current version of the course, we ask students to identify the theoretical frameworks that could answer their questions about data provided as part of a class data set. This assignment comes at the end of the semester, usually after students have had opportunities to engage with the data through close reading, summarizing, coding, and concept mapping. In other words, before our students begin the assignment, we want them to be very familiar with the data and the range of experiences it represents so they can approach it from a deeper analytic and theoretical perspective.

Students first identify an index case from the course data set. This case, following Timmermans and Tavory, can be a striking observation from the data, a contradiction people must reconcile, or an unfolding sequence of actions that reflect what's at stake in the situation (2022). The index case anchors further empirical analysis of the data and the analytic narrative that will develop. These cases can be excerpts that capture the most common patterns in the data or edge cases that represent extreme or unique perspectives and experiences.

From there, students use their index case to guide their analysis in terms of examining variation between cases and identifying patterns in the data. Next, they summarize a theoretical framework or perspective with which they want to analyze their data, starting with the index case, and explain why they chose it—what questions or insights did the index case spark, in terms of both the theory and the data? (Depending on the data and students' backgrounds, it might be necessary for us to offer ideas for potential theories.)

Course length constraints (we are working within eight-week terms) usually mean we don't ask our students to complete their analysis and write up any findings. Instead, we intend the assignment to encourage students to think about their data beyond mere description and consider what it can tell us about the social world.

Teaching theoretical perspectives

Several factors can make teaching theoretical perspectives a challenge in a qualitative research class. First, a short course won't allow you sufficient time to devote multiple class sessions to the complex content of different theoretical perspectives—on top of which, many students would likely consider such an allocation misaligned with their hopes or expectations for a methods course. Second, public health students often come from diverse backgrounds and may have different levels of comfort with various theoretical perspectives. This diversity of experience can make it very difficult to know which theoretical perspective(s) to use as illustrative examples.

For a semester-long class with more advanced students, you might take the approach suggested by Kawulich (2016). Dedicate the first few sessions to having students identify the substantive and formal theories in which they are interested and that they will use to guide their work as the class progresses. Kawulich provides a broad list of theories at the beginning of the course and has each student give a brief instruction to one theory as part of the class sessions. She recommends having students write up a summary handout for the rest of the class, one that includes the theory's originator, the questions typically associated with the theory, typical methods, and how the theory tends to be used. In Kawulich's experience, this approach engages students with the connections between theory and research and, by the end of the course, helps students develop a useful reference for future study planning. We haven't yet had a course that allows us this much time for theoretical consideration, but we can see that it's likely quite engaging!

Depending on your students' exposure, Kawulich's approach is likely to be too challenging. We've found public health students to be generally familiar with psychological frameworks (e.g., transtheoretical model, theory of planned behavior, health belief model, social cognitive theory) that that explore a participant's inner mental processes (intentions, motivations, self-efficacy). And, to the extent that students see these as the universe of possible explanatory models, the questions that they ask, the methods they employ, and the interpretation in which they engage may be limited. You might have to help students engage with other theoretical perspectives—those grounded in sociology, anthropology, economics, or gender studies, to name a few. This takes time, though, and is not really the focus of a methods class.

It is ideal if you can situate your qualitative methods class within a curriculum that includes complementary classes that expose students to a variety of the theoretical perspectives used in public health. In this scenario, you will be able to presume your students' familiarity with such perspectives and can use them without further explanation in your own class. However, you are more likely to be teaching students from a range of different backgrounds and with a variety of exposure to theoretical perspectives. In this case, you may need to cover the perspectives at least briefly and ask students to draw on what they do already know, even if that knowledge is incomplete.

Theorizing your analysis

Getting students to think about analysis in a qualitative course is another important time to engage with theory. (We discuss teaching analytic approaches and making sense of data in Chapter 6.) When it comes time to discuss analysis, we find that it is possible to provide and use, for illustrative purposes, one theory as an example everyone can use. Say, for example, that you are teaching qualitative data analysis. You might have your students read a foundational article or two (or even just extracts) on a concept such as therapeutic citizenship (a biopolitical concept linked to rights to medical knowledge and access to care/therapy). You could then have the students consider interview transcripts or other data through this lens. If you're teaching data collection approaches, you could develop exercises in which students write interview questions that reflect their theoretical perspective and answer questions that engage with core concepts from this perspective.

Alternatively, you could have students bring in theoretical frameworks they learned in other courses and apply those to their analytical work in your class. This approach only works if you know that your students have taken courses that covered theoretical perspectives; the advantage is that you can build upon the theory with which your students are already familiar. You can also build some theoretical exposure or exploration into your course through instructor-directed readings or by letting the students identify their own theoretical interests.

Summary

Theory and methods go hand in hand. A good qualitative methods course will also show students how theory shapes decisions about methods and the overall approach to a qualitative study. There are a lot of ways you can engage students with theory, and none of them are right or wrong (or necessarily easy). Introductory students may need nothing more than examples of how theory can influence decisions about the constructs you choose to study, along with sampling, analysis, and other variables. Advanced students can find grappling with theory a meaningful way to grow as a qualitative researcher and produce high-quality, theoretically driven, consistent research. Our sessions on the theoretical underpinnings of qualitative approaches—and especially our sessions on epistemology—have been some of the most influential for many of our students. They remember their "Aha!" moments from learning about epistemology or how to use a theoretical perspective to shape their approach to a study. As teachers, we have appreciated the ways we can help our students think differently. We encourage you to see theory as both a key element and potentially a highly engaging element of the course for your students!

4

Teaching Qualitative Study Design

When designing a qualitative research course, it's tempting to jump straight into methods without spending time getting students to think about all of the elements necessary for a good qualitative study. By prioritizing how we'll teach our students to think about collecting and analyzing qualitative data, we can too easily skip over critical questions about *why* we do this work in the ways that we do, as well as how we organize our overall approach to implementing a qualitative study.

In our experience, most students come to a qualitative methods course having had some exposure to research design instruction in their public health training. The challenge is that research design classes in public health often focus heavily on good *quantitative* study design principles and either wrongly assume that the same principles apply to qualitative studies or relegate qualitative design-specific considerations to a single lecture. In your qualitative methods course, you will likely need to at least revisit study design principles as they apply to qualitative methods, and you may need to introduce such principles entirely.

In essence, because public health students will likely be familiar with general quantitative study design, we need to call appropriate attention to the idea that the structure of qualitative research is usually—and appropriately—quite distinct. Researchers must make many decisions before they begin collecting data, many of which may differ from the approach one would take for a quantitative study. As a starting point, we must ensure that our research question is one that qualitative methods can answer. It's no use trying to

Teaching Qualitative Research in Public Health. Katherine Clegg Smith et al., Oxford University Press.
© Oxford University Press (2026). DOI: 10.1093/9780197662472.003.0004

shoehorn a quantitative question into a qualitative study design shoe; you'll get sore methodological feet and disappointing results, as Figure 4.1 illustrates! Other practical considerations include where research will occur, who will be included as participants and over what period, and what effect the research is intended to have.

In Chapter 1, we discussed the overarching principles of qualitative research, including some ideas of naturalistic design and centering participants' own words and perspectives. With this chapter, we consider how to turn these principles into study structure and how to teach qualitative study design considerations. This chapter offers guidance on both the conceptual and practical considerations that students need to consider both before they embark on a qualitative project and throughout the process.

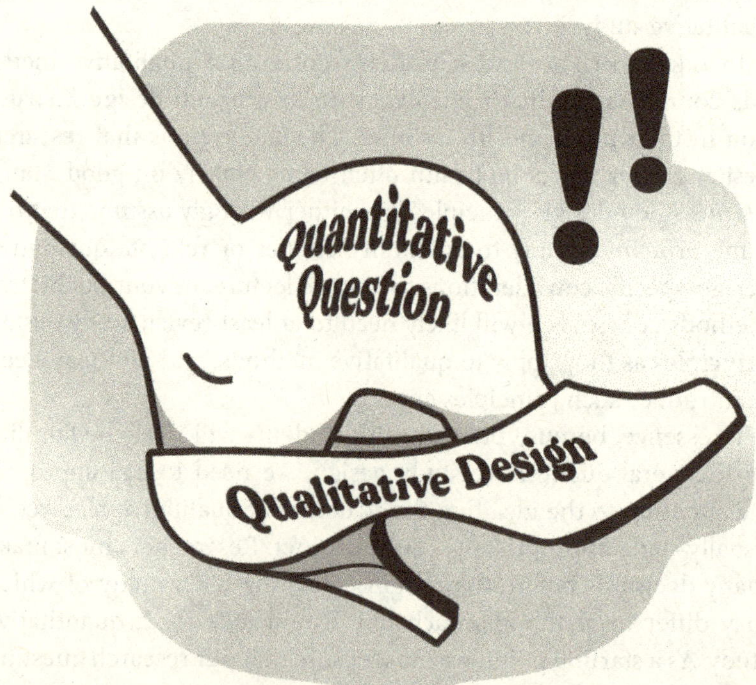

Figure 4.1 The study design needs to fit the research question

Asking qualitative questions

We start with the words of Michael Quinn Patton (2002): "Purpose is the controlling force in research. Decisions about design, measurement, analysis, and reporting all flow from purpose. Therefore, the first step in a research process is getting clear about purpose" (p. 213). A key starting point for students, in addition to considering their topic of interest, is to consider what kinds of pertinent research questions can be answered through qualitative methods. A common misunderstanding of qualitative research is that it is a means of gathering the same kinds of data as quantitative research, but quickly and on a smaller scale. A primary goal of any foundational qualitative research class should be addressing this misunderstanding wherever it is found. Qualitative research is not just small, quick quantitative research, nor is it a pilot test for quantitative research. Rather, it is fundamentally different: *qualitative research answers different questions than quantitative research.* The key is to know enough about each method, and the types of research questions they are designed to answer, to make a good decision. Box 4.1 provides some examples that can be used as analogies for matching the research question to the method.

Box 4.1 Tips and tricks: Matching the method to the question

We believe that any qualitative course in public health should include an explicit discussion of the fact that, when evaluating qualitative and quantitative research, one is not better or worse than the other. They are different approaches; each is best suited to particular research questions. We illustrate this point by getting students to think about two versions of something, each of which is distinct and good, and serves specific purposes. For example, you might consider horses (e.g., a racehorse versus a plow horse), cars (a minivan versus a convertible), or shoes (snow boots versus running

continued

> **Box 4.1** *continued*
>
> ---
>
> shoes). We reiterate that for any of these examples, one of the options is not better than the other, but one is better suited for any given task. The point is that no one would be well served by only one of the examples all the time. The task at hand is always what determines which item is the best choice.

Research questions that lend themselves to qualitative methods are typically nondirectional and based on naturalistic inquiry in which the researcher, rather than manipulate or intervene, observes and listens to understand. Such questions may, however, be applied to evaluations of clinical trials or implementation of programs and policies that are themselves interventional. In general, qualitative research questions seek to understand processes; do not seek to impose control; are highly attentive to context; focus on how people experience a phenomenon and the meaning they ascribe to it; and are open to complexity, ambiguity, and contradiction.

There are several ways to help students develop qualitative questions. For introductory students, you might start by explaining that qualitative research is often best suited for "How?" and "Why?" questions, whereas quantitative research is positioned to answer, "How many?" "Who?" or "When?" questions. You can note that qualitative research questions are ones that must be answered through words and explanations, while quantitative questions may be answered through numbers. You can then present students with a specific public health problem and ask them to develop both qualitative and quantitative research questions on this topic. Students often find template language helpful, such as "Describe," "Explore," and "Understand," in contrast to more quantitatively oriented questions such as "Affect," "Influence," "Impact," "Determine," and "Cause." (These discussions are great for "Think-Pair-Share" exercises.)

A second exercise may be to provide students with examples of specific qualitative and quantitative goals or with questions from your own research or from published literature. In this case, ask students to discuss why qualitative methods are better for answering one set of questions and quantitative methods better for another. A more advanced version of this exercise involves having students use quantitative questions to formulate a research question on the same topic that would be better answered with qualitative methods.

Finally, we encourage you to be creative! One idea would be to ask students to write a commercial that sells qualitative research to quantitative/biomedical researchers. Their commercial should communicate why qualitative research provides useful information impossible to get with quantitative methods. Or ask students to pretend they are a therapist with a client: what could they learn if they asked only quantitative questions, and what if they asked only qualitative questions?

Regardless of your approach, it is critical that, before you move to data collection and analysis, your students have a good sense of the kinds of research questions best suited to qualitative methods and which questions qualitative research cannot appropriately address.

Emergent design

Qualitative research often embraces an emergent design. (This method is also known as an iterative approach.) Qualitative public health researchers start with a plan for their study but remain open to changing different elements of their plan based on what they uncover in the field. Though they may be transformative, such changes don't potentially undermine a qualitative study. As qualitative researchers, we want and need to go where the data take us in order to best answer our question(s). We move between theory, data, and methods, revising our questions and methods as new information is revealed. Embracing an emergent design approach allows these changes to happen in an informed, intentional way.

Sometimes students conclude that an emergent and flexible design is the same thing as no study design. This is not the case! One strategy for teaching students about emergent design in qualitative research is to present them with case studies in which changes were made to initial plans based on either research conditions or emergent findings, then discuss how these changes either strengthened or undermined the study. Similarly, a creative strategy you might use to get students thinking through their choices when the right one isn't apparent until they're in the field is a "choose-your-own-adventure" activity. Put your students into groups and give them a brief overview of a research proposal—the main question, setting, data collection methods, and intended sample. Then, in five-minute intervals, give them three or four emergent factors to consider, along with the decision of whether to retain or modify their initial plan (and, if the latter, how they would modify it). At the end of the exercise, have each group (or a sample of them, depending on the size of the class) present their modifications and rationales to the class. This activity can help demonstrate the pros and cons of sticking to the original plan.

Depth versus breadth

Identifying a specific research question is critical for any study. We find that students frequently start with questions that are too broad to be addressed in a single study. In this instance, one key teaching goal is defining a reasonable research question to answer within a specific qualitative study design. While qualitative methods can offer in-depth perspective on a topic, gaining such a perspective is only possible if the scope of consideration is appropriate to the specific question *and* to the available resources—including time, finances, and human capacity.

In addition to the resources, determining study scope should also reflect the goals for the study in terms of its applicability and impact. Some students who are new to qualitative work find it challenging that qualitative research is usually not intended to generate findings applicable to an entire population. Indeed, the importance of context and a detailed, situated understanding of phenomena means that many findings are not immediately applicable beyond the specific setting or population within which a study was conducted. But this is hardly a limitation of a given study—it is one product of the way that the research is conducted, particularly when it is conducted well. In addition to its specific utility, knowledge from qualitative studies can often be transferred to other scenarios on a theoretical or conceptual level (i.e., through theoretical generalizability).

To get students engaged with the scope question, you might switch things up: instead of starting with a question, begin with a general area of interest and provide some of the conditions and resources available for a study on this topic. When conducting this thought exercise, we have students work backward to refine the nature of the question it may be reasonable to ask. Box 4.2 and Figure 4.2 offer concrete guidance for how to estimate time and resource needs for student projects.

Box 4.2 Tips and tricks: Estimating time and resource needs for student projects

---

It is common for students to underestimate the time they'll need to conduct qualitative research. Considering the size and scope of questions relative to an estimated sample helps students understand what might be required to answer a given question in the context of available data sources. You can give students examples of research questions from published literature, dissertations, senior projects at your own institution, or from your own work. Reducing the scope of a question might involve narrowing the parameters of the sample population (e.g., focusing on a village or hospital instead of a region or hospital system) or scaling back the topic of the question itself (e.g., turning a question about childrearing into one on parental perspectives about food and nutrition during the elementary school years). In our experience, students benefit from a rough estimate of the data generation time associated with a single one-hour interview, which could be up to 20 hours. As voice recognition software becomes increasingly sophisticated, the allocation of resources to transcription (i.e., time and/or money) will be reduced. As of this writing, though, we all still need to set aside time for checking transcriptions against the original

continued

Box 4.2 *continued*

audio to make sure that they accurately reflect the recordings. The time associated with transcription is especially important when working with populations who have their own dialect or vocabulary that might not be picked up by machine transcription. We also note that time "saved" by using automated transcription or a transcription service means more time will be needed for data immersion and/or familiarization.

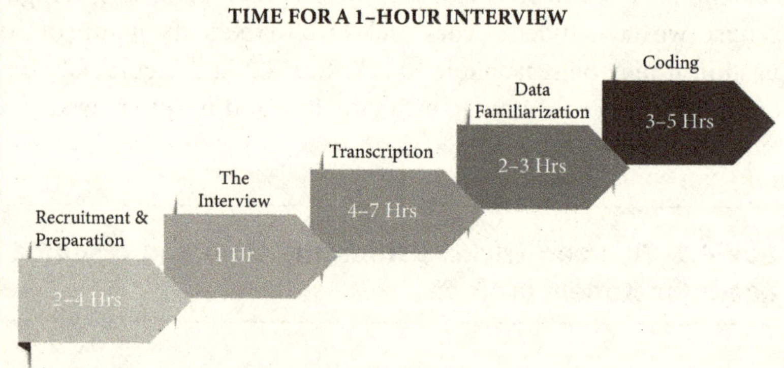

Figure 4.2   Estimated time associated with data curation from a one-hour qualitative interview

The study team

Your students' future research contexts will vary widely. Some will collect, manage, analyze, and write up the data alone; others may be members of a large international research team with a full complement of senior investigators, on-the-ground field staff, and data collectors. And some of them will experience both opportunities. Creating opportunities for your students to consider who they'll work with, what their and others' roles will be, and how to work in teams will help prepare them for the many forms that independent research can take. Teamwork has benefits both practical (like getting work done) and substantive (like having different perspectives and positionalities enrich the interpretive work). However, team-based work also invites complexity—particularly with work that is creative and highly interpretative. Not every team member needs to play the same role; teams often work best when each member's strengths combine in a complementary way. We bring our own experiences with solo and team research into our class discussions and ask students to share any team research experiences they may have had. While most students will be new to qualitative methods, we've also had several students with considerable prior experience doing qualitative research—even with no/minimal formal training, which is not something we recommend.

Sampling

Sampling is a key area in which good qualitative work requires something different than the quantitative approach. For the latter, we generally favor purposive over random sampling. Students need to understand why we use nonrandom sampling so they can construct strong samples for their own studies, justify their decisions to their peers and their audiences, and make informed assessments of others' studies.

Box 4.3 Tips and tricks: Explaining information-rich cases and purposive sampling

---

Random sampling is almost never the right approach for a qualitative study. We use an example of a carburetor to emphasize that sampling should always be related to the study's goal and objectives—recall the importance of selecting the right tool for a given job. To help students understand why random sampling is not always the best approach, we share a picture of a carburetor—yes, the car part. Then we ask the class,

continued

Box 4.3 *continued*

"If our research aim were to understand how a carburetor works, who would we sample?" The students will inevitably suggest interviewing auto mechanics or laypeople—a mechanically inclined uncle, perhaps—who happen to know a lot about cars. After a few suggestions, we respond, "I thought the gold standard was a random sample. Why wouldn't we select people at random from the general population?" Now, your students are ready for you to lead a class discussion about *why* a random sample is indeed the gold standard for many quantitative studies, but not usually qualitative ones. In quantitative research, the sample seeks representation and generalizability of a phenomenon in a population. The purpose of qualitative research, by contrast, is often understanding and contextual richness. Thus, a study's sampling approach should always be related to the study's objectives and goal. We return to the carburetor example throughout our courses—it's a memorable image, and we find it can be a powerful tool for challenging the belief that all good sampling is random sampling. From there, we bring up information-rich cases and alternate ways to do purposive sampling.

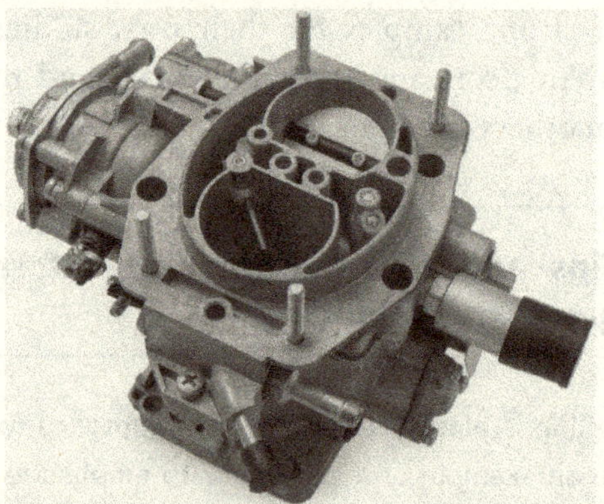

Figure 4.3 Photo of a carburetor for illustrative purposes (iStock.com/Phantom1311)

We find that the concept of sampling people who are information-rich makes sense to most students, once they hear it explained. However, many students then apply the concept to their own areas of interest and find it difficult to either identify those who might be information-rich for a given topic or how to recruit them. It may well be the case that when you're preparing for a study, the most information-rich participants might not be in plain sight. Just as qualitative studies generally follow an emergent design, sampling often evolves iteratively. Box 4.3 and Figure 4.3 provide our carburetor example for getting students to realize that a random sample is not always the best approach, while Box 4.4 and Figure 4.4 describe our detective analogy for explaining an iterative approach.

Box 4.4 Tips and tricks: Using the detective analogy to explain iterative sampling

---

A good way to engage the class in a consideration of iterative sampling is to either start with a picture of your favorite fictional detective—perhaps Hercule Poirot, Nancy Drew, or Sherlock Holmes—or have the class share their favorites. Then, ask your students how these detectives select who to sample when answering their research question: "Whodunit?" Detectives don't take random samples from the general population; in fact, at the beginning of a mystery, they often don't know who they should be speaking to at all! Instead, detectives work with whatever information they have at first. Then, they speak with whomever makes the most sense. That person suggests some clues, which leads the detective to speak with other people who provide more clues. As the detective pieces the information together, they may end up questioning people with whom they never thought to talk. The detective analogy is iterative sampling in action. As we learn more and more and can start answering our research questions, we may shift our sample or our entire sampling approach.

continued

Box 4.4 *continued*

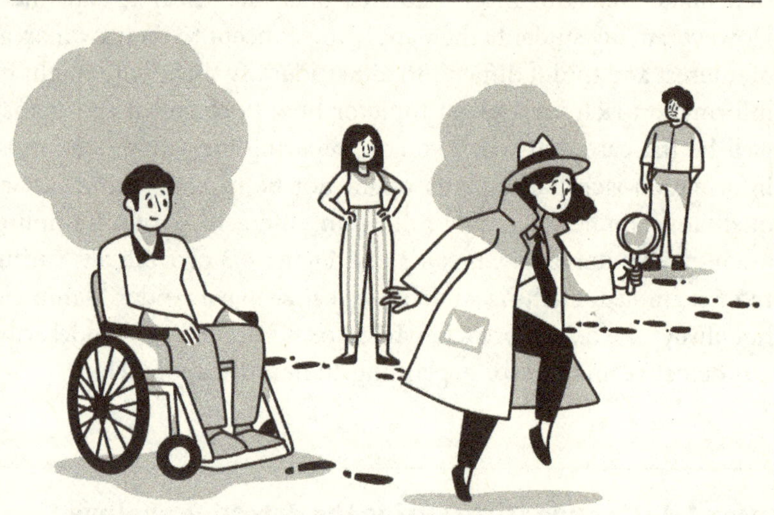

Figure 4.4 Iterative sampling involves building on what you learn from each participant

Of course, there is more to sampling than just finding information-rich cases. Patton's (2002) *Qualitative Evaluation and Research Methods* has an excellent list of purposive sampling approaches: maximum variation, homogenous, typical case, deviant case, snowball, and theoretical sampling. As an exercise, you might give the class a research topic and ask them to describe who they would sample using each of these different sampling strategies—and what the different approaches would mean for the ultimate analysis.

Sample size is another essential element of sampling. If qualitative methods professors had a dollar for every time a student asked them, "How many people do I need to interview?" or "How many focus groups do I need to do?" we would be a rich group of folks. Box 4.5 and Figure 4.5 provide our Goldilocks example for coming to the "just right" sample size.

Box 4.5 Tips and tricks: Using Goldilocks as an example of ideal qualitative sample size

In Goldilocks and the Three Bears, Goldilocks finds balance and things that are "just right"—not too big or too small, not too hot or too cold. You can use Goldilocks (or her methodologically inclined cousin, "Quali-locks") as a metaphor to illustrate that qualitative samples should be neither too big nor too small, but just right for getting the information you need to answer your research question with the least amount of data collection.

- **Too small**: does not achieve informational redundancy or theoretical saturation.
- **Too big**: cannot manage and facilitate the deep, case-oriented analysis that is the hallmark of qualitative research; participants are burdened needlessly.
- **Just right**: get the most information from the most limited data collection possible.

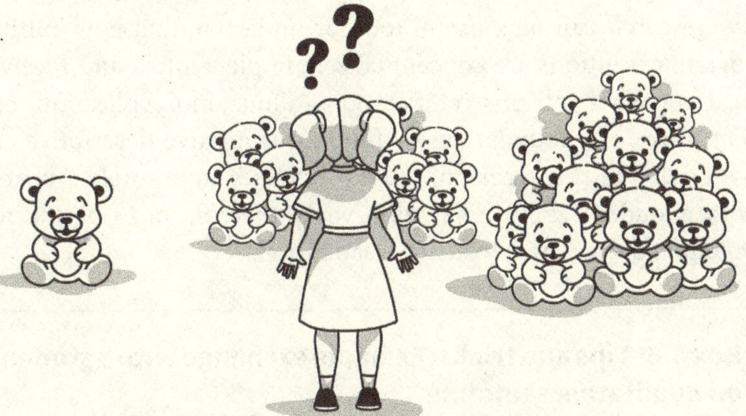

Figure 4.5 Quali-locks is trying to determine which sample size is "just right"

Qualitative researchers don't have power calculations to tell us that we've gathered enough data to answer a question. Saturation is an alternative concept that is used in qualitative research to aid in determining the ideal number of interviews, focus groups, or observations you'll need to answer a given question. The idea is to be mindful of when you start hearing the same responses repeatedly. The point beyond which a researcher is less and less likely to learn any new information that informs the research question(s) is the point at which the sample is becoming saturated. From here, the researcher should try to fill any remaining gaps in their knowledge and insight and then stop collecting data. Essentially, saturation can be interpreted as having the data necessary to answer all the elements of your research questions.

Given how exploratory some qualitative research is, there will be instances in which the universe of people or circumstances that can inform the topic is so small or specific that every case can—and should—be included in a study. We see this, for example, in studies that examine new policies and with research into innovative programs or novel clinical approaches to treatment. Qualitative research can be a useful tool for understanding how cutting-edge interventions are conceptualized, implemented, and received in a way that informs intervention rollout and replication, and that provides a foundation for future quantitative descriptive and hypothesis-testing research. Box 4.6 provides an example exchange with a student about a situation when there seem to be too few potential participants to achieve saturation.

Box 4.6   Tips and tricks: Example exchange with a student on qualitative sampling

---

Student: My dissertation will examine how a specific policy is being implemented in my state. Other states are showing interest in this policy, and I want to understand how the policy is being used by front-line implementers. My preliminary conversations with partners on the ground suggest that, while there was a lot of attention to the process of passing this law, not much has happened in the two years since its enactment. The exception is a suburban county where the local health officer charged a deputy health officer with overseeing implementation and set aside some funds to support this work. The team overseeing things has three people. This is not enough people to constitute a sample or reach saturation, right? What do I do?

Possible faculty response: Qualitative research should include the sources that can best inform the research. It sounds like your information-rich sources will be only a few people, but maybe not as few as you think. In addition to the team of three, you might also want to interview the health commissioner and the deputy health commissioner. Beyond those five people, are there any partner agencies or organizations involved who can inform your research questions? Are there any other sources of information (other than people) that can inform your research questions? Think about direct observation and document review, for example. And regardless of whether those possibilities pan out, this may be a time to include the universe of people and sources who can inform your research questions. To fully answer your research question, you may need to interview those handful of informants more than once. They may direct you to documents that can help you understand the implementation work they are doing that will further inform your research questions. Regardless of the details of the data you collect, working in this space will give you the chance to explore this topic deeply with the few people who are at its forefront.

Saturation is only possible with a truly iterative approach to data collection and analysis, such that the researcher is fully engaged with their data throughout. Without analyzing data as it is collected, it's impossible to know when saturation has been reached and whether additional sources of information are needed, or when additional follow-up interviews with informants to achieve saturation or round out their understanding of a phenomenon may be warranted. Familiarity with the data and learning from the field are also critical to gaining confidence about sampling and saturation. This is something that often comes with experience, although the classroom is a place to establish the skills for engaging in those processes. You might have your students read published studies that explain how their authors made sampling and saturation decisions, complete in-class exercises that allow them to work with data that are responsive to a qualitative research question, or share firsthand examples from established researchers who have managed these issues in their own studies.

An iterative approach to sampling and sample size must be balanced with the practical considerations necessary for study planning—things like timelines, IRB review, and available funding. In general, we recommend that students slightly *overestimate* the sample size they'll need at the start of a study (while keeping it within realistic limits). Research funds and ethical approval can usually accommodate overestimates much better than underestimates. It's also always easier to complete a study early than to ask for more money and time!

We find that advanced students are often nervous about saturation. They wonder whether they'll know when they've reached it and how they can be sure they wouldn't find more information if they talked with just one more person. One way to address their anxiety is to direct them back to their research question and remind them that the goal of research is communicating findings to others. When the researcher can make claims based on their data, stand behind their work, and answer their question based on the principles of saturation, they should feel confident. True, there's always some chance that interviewing one more person would have added something new. But if students believe their goal is to provide a rigorous, situated understanding of a phenomenon or topic and not an ironclad law of nature, they should remember that they can, if needed, change their understanding based on new information.

One idea that complements saturation is information power. Malterud and colleagues (2016) have suggested that where qualitative interview studies are concerned, the more information in the sample that is relevant for the actual study, the fewer participants are needed. They propose that sample size depends on the following five factors:

1. **The study's aim**. The narrower the study aim, the smaller the necessary sample size.
2. **Sample specificity**. The necessary sample size will decrease as its participants' knowledge and experience increase.
3. **Use of established theory**. The more theory you apply to focus the analysis, the smaller the sample size you'll need.
4. **Quality of dialogue**. Stronger dialogue between researcher and participants reduces the size of the needed sample.
5. **Analysis strategy**. A single-case, descriptive analysis will require a smaller sample size than a cross-case analysis that seeks to compare patterns across cases.

The concept of information power aligns with our own experience; we've also found that rich data can require a smaller sample size than a large data set comprised of thin data in order to meet a study's aims. Information power can help students grasp the nuances of sampling in qualitative research, as it captures well the notion that all potential interviewees will not yield the same quality of insight and should be weighed accordingly. (Of course, getting the right data sources to answer your questions is a whole other challenge.)

Recruitment

Once a researcher selects *who* they plan to include as study participants, they must also figure out *how* to reach them. This is the difference between sampling and recruitment. Ensuring that your course design considers the philosophical underpinnings of sampling and the practical considerations of recruiting that sample creates a balanced curriculum, one in which students can both understand the thinking behind the work and be confident in their own ability to do it. For those "how" skills, recruitment is a specific form of access. The points we make below about people can also apply to entry into important spaces or acceptance into relevant communities.

Recruitment usually starts with practical questions:

- Where are your potential participants?
- How can you reach them?

As we alluded to above, purposive sampling strategies may help us select participants based on characteristics that may not be publicly visible or easy to sample. We want information-rich participants—but how do we identify them? How can we determine which people will be particularly thorough and thoughtful in their responses, engaged with our topics, adept at communicating their experiences to others, or comfortable sharing their experiences with the study team? How can theoretical sampling tell us which people might have a specific type of experience?

We've heard these questions from students for years. Reassuring them and giving them strategies for sampling through recruitment is critical to moving the class forward. For one thing, students need to consider how their recruiting mechanisms—community organizations, clinical service providers, social media, or community flyers, to name a few examples—will shape not only who they recruit to a study but the nature of participants' connection to it. Say there's an existing clinical trial or cohort study collecting quantitative data about attitudinal, behavioral, or experiential questions; a qualitative study could use the quantitative data to select qualitative participants who meet certain characteristics. This may indeed be a highly effective and efficient way of identifying valuable participants. However, basing the sample on the trial's foundation will shape the nature of the data that the qualitative study generates, as well as its utility for answering qualitative research questions.

It's often useful to have students imagine precisely who they might be looking for in a study and to then have them think about how they might both find such people and give them an opportunity to participate. Doing so is also a good way for you to assess how your students are applying the course content and, if needed, to provide them with additional instruction on sampling for qualitative research.

One possible recruitment exercise is to give your students a sample research aim. Break them into groups of three or four and have them discuss how they would recruit individuals for this aim. Who can answer their question, and how will they find such individuals? Bring everyone back together so the groups can share feedback with the entire class and note the similarities and differences in their approaches. This exercise encourages reflection on the strengths and challenges of the different approaches and the class can collectively consider whether specific approaches, developed for specific groups, would be appropriate for others.

For example, some groups of people are harder for public health researchers to identify and contact than others. It's also the case that, within any group, some people will be more comfortable talking than others, and that some groups will simply be more challenging to reach. But that doesn't mean that you shouldn't try talking to those challenging groups and the quieter individuals. Those who are less outgoing or talkative may also have specific and distinct insights that are important for your research. It's imperative that qualitative studies include marginalized people and communities (just as it is for quantitative studies). Recruitment strategies emphasizing inclusivity and providing mechanisms for inclusive sampling are important to teach and essential for rigorous qualitative methods.

One way to locate those harder-to-reach individuals and communities is through snowball sampling. This technique is as much about recruitment as it is about sampling. In this type of sample, early participants recommend other people who they feel are information-rich or who have a specific set of characteristics, beliefs, or experiences prioritized by the study team. A snowball-generated sample will, by its very nature, not include members who are independent from one another. Snowball sampling is one example of a recruitment method used and well-suited to qualitative research. We encourage you, however, to introduce snowball sampling but also go well beyond this method and invite your class to consider a range of inclusive recruitment scenarios.

Of course, if you ask students to conduct a qualitative study as part of your course, then teaching recruitment means they'll have to figure out how to engage participants for their study. This type of assignment has the benefit of seeing—up close and personal—all the real-world challenges of recruitment! In addition to learning that posting a community flyer usually does not result in a flood of interest, our students discover regularly that participants don't always show up for a scheduled interview, even in situations when the students think they made a connection with a potential participant during recruitment outreach.

Teaching about recruitment may be a place to bring up issues of power, positionality, and reflexivity. We've worked with clinicians who offered to recruit their patients into our research studies, telling us, "No problem! They'd be happy to do that for me!" However, keep in mind the established relationships and power dynamics at play in such a recruitment scenario. An example like this is a teachable opportunity, one where your students can contemplate how to ensure their recruitment strategies are ethical and do not create opportunities for coercion due to unequal power dynamics.

Community engagement and embeddedness

The relationship between the researcher and the community or individuals who participate in the study can and will affect recruitment coordination, the nature of the research questions that can be asked and answered, the type of data that can be collected, the rigor of the data and the strategies that may be needed to enhance rigor, and how the data will be disseminated and used at the end of the study. Gold's (1958) classic typology of the four researcher roles in participant observation ranges along a continuum from complete participant to complete observer (see Chapter 5). It can be very helpful to walk through each distinct observational stance with the class and have them discuss, in small groups, the implications of each role for different research questions in different settings. Guiding discussions that center questions about informed consent, the data collection options available to each role, and the implications of the kinds of information the roles may yield can help students appreciate the many ways to approach qualitative design—and how design decisions affect what a study finds.

Gold's typology defines different options for relationships with research participants or communities, but how these typologies are applied often depends on partnerships. (This is particularly true when the researcher is an outsider.) The extent to which a research project is either inspired by a partnership with a nonacademic agency or organization or is the inspiration for establishing a partnership has implications for the options available to the researcher in Gold's framework. The implications of partnerships for study design decisions are a particularly important consideration for advanced students. A doctoral seminar designed to help students develop their dissertation proposals could include examples of partner engagement in research from experienced faculty members, detailing the ways that those partnerships began and how they evolved to include research. By discussing partnership navigation with the faculty members themselves, students can better envision how partnered research may figure into their own work—either with their dissertations or later in their careers.

For such classroom content, the community-based participatory research literature and other participatory action research methods offer helpful instruction on involving community organizations as research partners, including for qualitative research. These approaches share the recognition that research happens in communities, rather than a controlled environment. They prioritize impacted individuals and communities playing a key role in decisions about how the research is conceived, conducted, presented, and disseminated. Community partnership discussions can become opportunities to understand power, control, who has a say in conducting the research, how the research portrays communities, and what happens with the findings. Such discussions can also be opportunities for students to consider the type of institution with which they are affiliated (e.g., a predominately white-serving institution, a minority-serving institution), how their institutional identity affects potential community-affiliated research partners' understanding of the research, and the influence of these dynamics on their approach to the work.

You may also, depending on your course structure, have a chance to explore these dynamics through field-based coursework. If you are partnering with community-based organizations to conduct qualitative projects in real time (as described in Chapter 2), you might ask your students to reflect on the nature of their partnerships and identify preconceptions about working with their community partners or how power and privilege may be affecting their work. The service-learning literature can offer supplemental reading and guidance for your students and your instruction. Service learning embraces the classroom as a venue for partnership, one in which the academic instructor and the community member are cocreators in partnered projects and course goals. Service-learning assignments should produce lessons for the students and products for the partner organization, and, as such, represent a chance for students to learn by doing.

We also note that the time researchers spend in the field affects the engagement with and relationship between both researchers and partners and researchers and participants. Field engagement in public health is typically shorter—by weeks or months—than other disciplines that use qualitative methods. Anthropologists, for example, may stay in the field or embedded within a community for years. More time in the field can mean more partner engagement in the substantive processes of study design, data collection and analysis, and dissemination of study findings. Regardless of the amount of field time, study designs that include participatory methods require intention consideration of the partner relationship throughout the study and often rely on partner investments in the planning of research. One way to illustrate this is to assign students to read a paper that used extended field engagement as well as one on findings from a brief period in the field. This allows students to compare and contrast the different research questions, methods, and findings from each. This exercise will provide an opportunity to reflect on the two very different scenarios in the context of their own research interests.

Data management

From the start, students need to plan for how they'll manage a study's data. Your course goals will determine whether you need to spend a lot of time on data management. In more advanced, practice-based courses, data management features prominently. We find that encouraging students to work backward and think first about the information they'll need for their analysis to be a helpful approach. Should they need demographic information about their participants, they learn they must collect it from the start. We encourage students to create data management procedures *before* they embark on data collection. We also talk about organizing data and sharing sample spreadsheets to help students track the steps of every interview: scheduling, conducting, transcribing, and coding. In essence, we've found that real-world examples of approaches used in other studies are the best way to learn.

Bringing it all together with a methodological approach

Methodologies are more closely related to the process of doing research and provide strategies or overall plans of action to inform the design of a qualitative study. We discussed methodologies as part of Crotty's (1998) framework. Creswell and Poth (2017) described five methodologies: ethnography, phenomenology, case study research, narrative research, and grounded theory. Each of these approaches provides an overall plan for framing research questions, selecting data collection methods, considering aspects of study rigor, and analyzing data to produce a final research product. Students often appreciate the clear and concise guidance that Creswell and Poth offer in their book.

We tend to start with grounded theory, as we find that some students have heard of it. Occasionally, students share that they think the term is synonymous with qualitative research, and we then explain how this is not the case! Grounded theory, developed by Glaser and Strauss (1967), is not a theory unto itself, but a method used to develop midlevel theories—those theories that bridge higher-level concepts with empirical data to provide a conceptual understanding within a specific applied area. One good example of grounded theory in public health is Poteat et al.'s (2013) research to outline stigma in health care encounters for transgender adults. Grounded theory relies on inductive analysis, constructing codes and categories directly from the data instead of from preexisting theories or ideas. It uses the constant comparative method and theoretical sampling to build up to these theories and advance theory during the iterative steps of data collection and analysis. Because its analytical steps are so clear and detailed, we often teach grounded theory in our advanced data analysis courses as it provides a process for students to follow.

Grounded theory is, however, far from the only qualitative methodology out there. Many students have also heard of ethnography. Ethnography has a much longer history than grounded theory, but it is more difficult to connect to specific techniques and methods. Ethnography is usually characterized by a focus on shared culture and the use of participant observation, among other techniques, to immerse the researcher in a given culture and the systems that structure it. Case study research is another methodological approach that generally uses multiple data collection methods to describe one or more "cases." A case is a bounded system in time and place (e.g., an event, an experience, or an organization) chosen because of the impossibility of separating the case from its context and the value of the case to understanding a phenomenon of interest. Narrative research, by contrast, focuses on the stories that people tell and how they tell them. Finally, phenomenology centers the subjective, lived experience of a specific phenomenon, such as living with a chronic illness.

Different methodologies will shape the approach to a given research question—and why one approach could be selected over another. Often, we prompt students to describe how they might use each methodology to study a sample topic. In one course, the lecture on methodologies often coincides with the Super Bowl; when this happens, we put up pictures of the two football teams playing that year and ask how a study of the Super Bowl would look different if approached from each methodology. A narrative study might focus on the narrative arcs that each team uses to describe their journey to the big game, highlighting how the different characters are portrayed, the moments of epiphany or turning points, and how the narratives serve specific purposes—what the teams highlight or leave out, and whose interests they served by doing so. An ethnographic study might embed the researcher within the locker rooms to study the culture of each team. We've also used other current events, such as presidential elections, as examples, and find that it can sometimes be useful to engage with examples outside of public health so students can brainstorm more freely. However, there are plenty of public health topics that you could use for this exercise as well. For example, if you chose the topic of sports injuries, students might propose a narrative study to examine individual injury and care-seeking trajectories, or an ethnographic study to understand different sports teams' approaches to managing potential concussions.

In advanced classes, we go into more depth about these methodologies and highlight areas where a single methodology features divergent paths. When we present the history of grounded theory, we note that Glaser and Strauss ultimately took the theory in different directions during its development and point out there are both objectivist and constructivist approaches to grounded theory. Furthermore, these classes let us explain the areas where the methodologies sometimes are more similar than different: constructivist approaches to phenomenology and grounded theory could have more in common than two grounded theory studies with different epistemological approaches.

We also want to ensure that our students understand what these methodologies are and are not. The five methodologies build on rich traditions of scholarship. Drawing upon these traditions to inform a qualitative study's design means that a researcher can build upon the ideas of many bright thinkers before them. Following a tradition can also help researchers justify their study design decisions. Creswell and Poth's five traditions are not, however, the only options for a qualitative study. Indeed, many students who feel that none of these options fit their research question are relieved to learn that one need not explicitly choose a methodology at all! Many qualitative studies, particularly in public health, are conducted without defining an explicit methodological frame.

We believe students should be taught the importance of being able to explain their qualitative study design choices. Design choices should fit together in that they contain complementary assumptions and make sense. Sometimes, tapping into a methodological tradition can unite the design of a qualitative study under a more holistic approach; in other instances, students may want to make design choices that don't fit quite as neatly. From our perspective, so long as the students can justify their choices, this approach is fine! We also encourage students to be precise when they describe what they did and did not do with their design decisions. For example, students may find it helpful to note that they used specific analytic techniques drawn from grounded theory, such as line-by-line coding, even if they do not want to label the study a grounded theory study. The critical thinking encouraged by these discussions will serve your students well in their qualitative training, and in their public health pursuits generally.

Summary

It's crucial in designing a qualitative research course to emphasize foundational elements beyond just methods. Students should understand why qualitative methods are distinct from quantitative ones, ensuring they can appropriately frame research questions that qualitative methods can effectively address. This involves revisiting study design principles specifically tailored to qualitative research, which often differ significantly from quantitative approaches. Practical considerations such as research context, participant selection, and intended impact also need careful planning to ensure students grasp the holistic approach required for successful qualitative studies in public health. In the next chapter, we start to unpack how we engage students in these decisions.

5

Teaching Qualitative Methods

This chapter addresses teaching interviews, focus groups, observation, and document analysis. Our goal is not to provide everything you could ever need to teach each approach—there are fantastic coursebooks on each particular data collection method, as well as great overview texts on qualitative methods. Instead, we describe how we approach teaching this material for different audiences or course objectives and offer an overview of the topics you might want to cover for each method.

Any qualitative course needs to convey certain essential information about key methods to prepare students to be critical consumers of study findings or to embark on their own research. To reinforce our guidance, we often ground our teaching content in our own experiences, as well as those of other researchers whom we see engaging in exemplary work. And while we seek to avoid giving directives, at times some students will look for hard-and-fast rules they can reference to know that they're doing it right.

Teaching qualitative methods with diverse learners

Students often come to a qualitative methods class with a vague understanding of the common qualitative data collection methods. They've likely heard of focus groups and qualitative interviews but are less likely to have heard of participant observation or considered the use of documents or artifacts as data. Regardless of the students' knowledge base, most instructors of qualitative courses

Teaching Qualitative Research in Public Health. Katherine Clegg Smith et al., Oxford University Press.
© Oxford University Press (2026). DOI: 10.1093/9780197662472.003.0005

will want to explain an array of approaches typically used in qualitative public health research, as well as help students know when and why to use specific methods for a given question or research scenario.

As we established in Chapter 2, your goal may or may not be to prepare your students to begin an actual study by the end of the course. Learning how to conduct qualitative research is an important motivator for many students enrolled in a qualitative course, but it's difficult for a single course to cover all the material students will need to know. It is good practice to outline your expectations clearly from the start and tailor classroom activities and other learning to them. And remember: **fostering an appreciation of qualitative approaches and building the capacity to conduct qualitative research are both worthwhile goals that require different approaches in the classroom.**

For your least-intensive or introductory courses, your goal may be to leave students with a general appreciation for the various qualitative data collection methods and how to use each one to answer public health questions. This may be all you can cover in the allotted time—and that's perfectly fine! With more intense courses and/or more experienced students, you may be able to create conditions in which students can get hands-on experience or even engage in conducting a qualitative research study. In this case, you'll need to provide them with not only an understanding of what qualitative research is but also how to do it—and how to do it well.

This distinction in course goals can be challenging because students are likely to want to get ready to undertake some qualitative work by the end of the course. This can be challenging if the course is brief, or if you include qualitative methods as only one part of a general social science research methods class. Qualitative methods may seem easy and intuitive—there is a common misconception that "it's just talking to people." On the contrary, significant training and practice are necessary to obtain useful data that can address important public health problems. Setting expectations for both yourself and students about what knowledge and skills they will acquire through the course is critical. You can develop your students' appreciation of qualitative methods in less-intensive courses by giving them examples of how such methods have been applied in practice. For examples, we tend to draw heavily on our own work and that of our colleagues, in addition to that of our students. Doing so allows us to talk authentically and candidly about development of research plans, what went well, the effect of the research, and what we would change if we had the chance. In courses where students won't get hands-on experience, these specific accounts can be particularly useful.

You can complement didactic content on the basics of qualitative research with demonstrations of and opportunities for students to engage in data collection. Engaged activities can build your students' practical skills and their capacity for conducting qualitative research before they undertake their first project. You might have a faculty member describe and demonstrate the different methods; you may also give your students space to try the methods themselves.

At a minimum, a qualitative research class in public health should include a discussion of interviews, focus groups, observation, and document/artifact research.

It may also be helpful to introduce specific methods from allied research approaches, such as participatory action research and arts-based methods. We have not included an overview of these methods here, although you may choose to incorporate them into your course.

The research question is critical in choosing a method

In designing our courses, we emphasize the importance of understanding that different research methods generate different types of data. Even students who begin our courses with some knowledge of different qualitative methods often don't know how to fit a method to a scenario. They also need guidance on what to do and how to know whether they did it correctly.

We further emphasize that qualitative methods are better suited to answer certain questions—or, as we put it, "The research question should determine the methods employed." As Box 5.1 illustrates, different questions ("jobs") require different methods ("tools") to answer them. When students tell us that they intend to "do a qualitative aim" for their dissertation proposal or that they want their master's capstone to involve qualitative analysis, we encourage them to flip the script and instead ask which methods would best answer their research question(s). To a teacher, this approach may seem obvious, but remember to make clear to your students that qualitative methods are of little use if the question is best served by quantification. If a study needs to establish "How many?" or "Are people more or less likely to?" then it is not best served through a qualitative approach no matter how much a student may want to "do a qualitative aim."

Furthermore, even if students do identify a qualitatively appropriate research question, they need to understand that each qualitative method produces a different type of data.

- Qualitative interviews generate responses to a researcher's specific questions or prompts.
- Focus groups generate discussion among people who have a common connection to an issue or topic.
- Observation or fieldwork produces notes on or recordings of naturally occurring events or interactions recorded by a specific researcher in a specific context.
- Working with documents or social artifacts results in the interpretation of socially relevant products or documents by a specific researcher or research team.

It is important to impart the understanding that different qualitative methods are good for collecting different types of data and answering different kinds of questions. Interviews aren't necessarily better than focus groups or observations; the fit with the question is key. A qualitative course should prompt students to consider the strengths and limitations of each data source relative to their questions of interest. The perfect tool for one job may be neither nimble, powerful, nor effective when applied to another.

Box 5.1 Tips and tricks: Choosing the right tool for the job

We use an exercise to illustrate the importance of alignment between question and method in which we present two very different versions of a high-quality object (e.g., an electric versus an acoustic guitar, a sports car versus a high-end minivan, or a raincoat versus a ski jacket) side-by-side. For example, Figure 5.1 presents the dilemma of which rental vehicle would make the most sense for the parent to rent, given the circumstances (lots of people, luggage, pets, etc.). We ask students to consider the circumstances that would lead them to choose one over the other. Is the same object always the best choice? What happens to the value of one when you choose it, and it turns out the other would have been better?

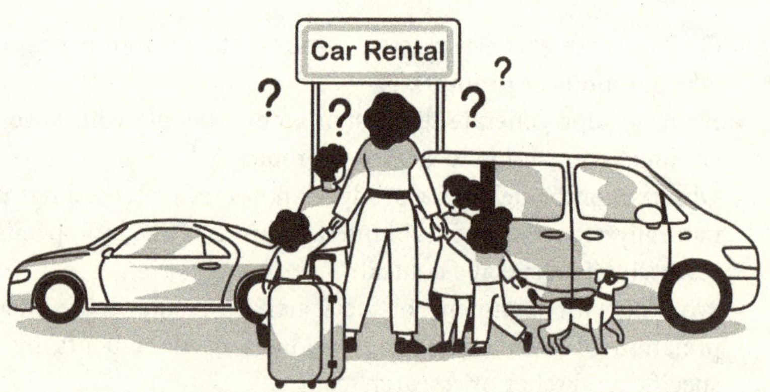

Figure 5.1 The choice of method depends on what is right for the job at hand

A related activity involves asking students to design a party menu for their 6-year-old niece or their 60-year-old father—the perfect menu for one might be terrible for the other. This activity can also be a memorable way to demonstrate how one option is better than the other only when you understand what you need your choice to do.

After introducing the methods, you might give your students a research question and have them pair up to discuss the strengths and limitations of applying a given method. For example, if you wanted to understand how dangerous or violent student behavior is dealt with in public high schools, what could you learn by doing the following:

- interviewing 20 teachers from a range of schools
- interviewing 20 people in school leadership positions
- analyzing school discipline policies or codes of conduct
- conducting focus groups with students from a range of schools
- observing in one or two schools for an extended period

Interviews

Interviews, and particularly in-depth or semi-structured interviews, are a core qualitative research method across many applied disciplines, including public health. Interviews allow you to ask open-ended questions that help you to understand how participants feel about a research topic or how they have experienced it.

As is often the case with some aspects of qualitative research, you may encounter students who begin your course with a rough idea of what a qualitative interview looks like. Even something like their familiarity with TV shows or podcasts that use an interview format may lead them to believe they understand the method and are ready to try their skills in the field. In this case, we have found it important to gently remind them that they are novices and that qualitative research is research and distinct from journalism or entertainment.

Qualitative interviewing is a skill developed through study, practice, and critical reflection; there is much to learn about this method in a qualitative course before one is ready for the field.

You may want your course to cover only the most basic concepts about qualitative interviews:

- What is a qualitative interview?
- What data are generated through such an interview?
- Why choose interviews over other qualitative methods?
- What kinds of questions do you ask?

Below, we outline these and other qualitative interview topics for the classroom, from basic to advanced concepts.

What is a qualitative interview?

We find that many students in introductory public health courses initially have a quantitative mindset. We therefore emphasize a qualitative interview's open-ended, dialogic nature: the exchange is a conversation, not a survey. Differentiating the approaches can be tricky, however, because the meaning of the word "interview" is context dependent. Researchers sometimes call a survey a "researcher-administered interview" if they want to indicate that data are collected through a researcher and not by the participant alone (e.g., self-administered on a computer). For a class exercise, you might watch a short clip of a qualitative interview and another of a researcher asking survey questions, then ask students to discuss the interactional styles and the data generated. In a course where students have a deeper background knowledge, you might discuss the history of qualitative interviews and their use for different purposes in different disciplines.

Once students understand what a qualitative interview is, they can explore the types of data these interviews generate and how they differ from other approaches to data collection.

How to structure an interview

When appropriate, as Figure 5.2 shows, we present qualitative interviews on a continuum of structure and control that ranges from unstructured (casual conversations that can happen, for example, over the course of an extended period of participant observation) to semi-structured (in which the interviewer has a set of topics to cover but the flexibility to ask specific questions around those topics) to structured (where there is a predetermined set of questions) and surveys (comprised of predetermined questions with predetermined and closed-ended answer choices). Each of these requires a different approach to the design of the interview guide (also sometimes known as a field guide). In fact, unstructured interviews may require no guides at all. Semi-structured interview guides may list just a few key topics or questions, while structured approaches will likely involve a complex list of tailored questions, discussion prompts, and instructions for reacting to specific responses. The nature of the interview structure will shape the data generated. A more loosely structured interview has a greater potential for more varied responses, which is both potentially generative and sometimes challenging for the researcher who may not be prepared for some of the responses provided.

We also teach the different phases of qualitative interviewing. One of the strengths of qualitative research is its flexibility, which allows the researcher to incorporate an iterative design (see Chapter 3). An iterative approach means that a study's first few interviews are often exploratory—with a goal of establishing which topics prompt people to provide useful data, or of identifying topics for inquiry that hadn't been considered by the research team. It's therefore possible that subsequent interviews will be more structured or intended to follow up on key topics and confirm findings from earlier interviews.

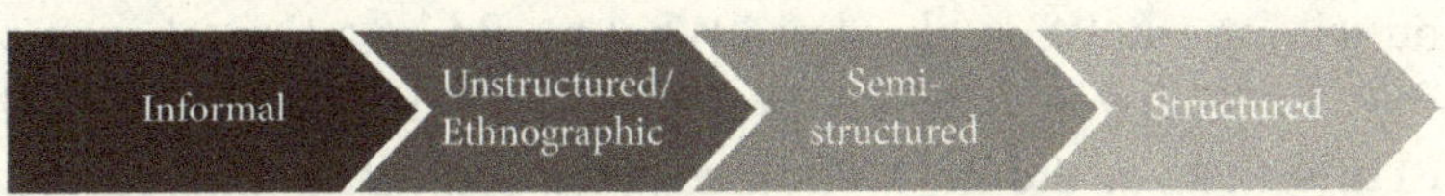

Figure 5.2 Qualitative interviews as a continuum of structure and control

It's also possible that every interview in a study will proceed with limited structure. It all depends on the study's goals.

There are many ways to structure an interview. A life history interview, to give just one example, is likely to be structured around life stages or milestone events, sometimes with a timeline to aid participants' memories. An interview structure and approach can also differ for follow-up interviews with the same participant. Specific goals of follow-up interviews may include:

- going deeper, with increasing focus
- building rapport and trust
- obtaining clarification
- testing ideas or interpretations
- addressing questions from your guide that were not covered in the first interview

When we introduce students to different types of interview questions, we also discuss how, at the beginning of an interview, it's usually a good idea to ask open-ended questions, so the participant can answer in their own way. We point out that when an interview is comfortable and conversational, a question that could be answered with a yes or a no usually will not be. Lest our students begin to think that there's nothing more to qualitative questioning than being open-ended, though, we discuss avoiding leading questions, techniques for probing and follow-up, and the range of question types that Spradley (2016) has categorized as descriptive, structural, and contrast questions.

As a class activity, you might develop a game that asks students to fit questions into Spradley's categories or to identify open-ended versus closed-ended questions. An assessment activity could be to ask students to generate an interview guide on a particular topic using three to five of Spradley's descriptive questions (e.g., "Could you tell me what X is like?" or "What would be a typical example of Y?" or "Can you walk me through everything that happened the last time that you did Z?"). The instructor would help the students to see how the goal of such questions is to elicit a body of language on a topic from the participants' perspective and lived experience, while imposing as little structure or assumptions as possible from the outside. These kinds of questions can lead to very extensive responses if rapport between the interviewer and interviewee is well established. The instructor might want to act as a surrogate respondent to demonstrate what the exchange might look like.

An alternative activity that might be an easier starting place for relatively novice students would be to present a set of leading questions and have students rephrase them into nonleading questions.

Interview questions can be organized into an interview guide. In addition to discussing the development of such a guide, we address the funnel approach to interview organization, which involves beginning an interview with broad, overarching questions before homing in on specific areas. Because students often conflate an interview guide with a survey instrument, an analogy can help them understand the difference: think of a survey instrument as the instructions for a piece of self-assembled furniture (where it is critical that every step be followed in order and as described) and a qualitative guide as a recipe for spaghetti sauce (because it's fine to allow for some improvisation, and where experienced professionals may rely very little on formal instructions). Box 5.2 provides one example classroom exercise that can help students understand the differences between surveys and interview guides and the types of data that each generates.

Box 5.2 Tips and tricks: Comparing surveys and semi-structured interviews

Objective: Helping students understand the differences between surveys and interview guides in terms of the types of data each generate and what makes them appropriate for data collection.

Begin with a brief overview of both data collection methods, along with the differences between structured surveys, semi-structured interviews, and unstructured interviews.

continued

> **Box 5.2** *continued*
>
> ---
>
> Next, give your students a sample survey and interview guide for the same topic. Divide the students into small groups and instruct them to analyze the types of data that could be generated from each method. Remind them to consider the advantages and disadvantages—including the richness, depth, and flexibility of data collection—of each approach.
>
> Finally, discuss as a class the circumstances that dictate the appropriateness of each method, based on research objectives and the type of data needed.

While drafting an interview guide can be an excellent assignment, grading it may prove challenging. It's relatively easy to grade on question style—e.g., Does the guide include open-ended questions?—but it is much harder to grade the quality of the content. We suggest several review components: peer feedback, instructor assessment, and peer assessment of the guide in action through an in-class mock interview. The mock interview is an especially helpful opportunity to refine questions—and, depending on the level of revisions, it may be further helpful for students to then assess the revised guide.

Speaking of refinement, we further emphasize that follow-up interview techniques are different than those for initial interviews. Because a follow-up should build upon the previous interview, the interviewer will generally want to reread the first interview and use it to develop new questions. They can look for important themes. Did issues come up repeatedly? Are there elements that have been oversimplified and require more detail, context, or nuance? The interviewer can also identify stories or narratives that may not have been fully explored. Follow-up interviews might be a good time to ask different types of questions—for example, structural or contrast questions (Spradley, 2016) that add to the foundation established in the original interview.

You can address follow-up interviewing techniques with a class exercise: assign students to read a portion of a transcript where the interviewee goes into considerable depth about a topic, then pauses. In class ask your students what questions they might ask next and discuss the various lines of inquiry. A homework exercise is another option: give your students a brief overview of one study's goals and an interview transcript from this study and have them generate topics they might bring up and interview questions they might ask in a follow-up interview.

Interview logistics

In an introductory or very low-intensity course, you may not discuss interview logistics at all; conducting qualitative interviews may simply not be a career goal for students enrolled in such a course. Beyond these, however, most courses will want to provide students with training in the nuts and bolts of conducting a qualitative interview.

The following paragraphs outline the elements of our instruction in interview logistics. We outline the aspects of the experience that all researchers should plan for and the issues likely to arise in the field. However, as interviewing is a somewhat personal, individual endeavor, we base our instruction in our own experience. And we model these individual aspects by keeping our logistics classes conversational—we raise key elements of quality data generation, present personal experiences, and invite questions.

Finding people and finding interview locations

We start at the very beginning, with interview recruitment and location. This is a great topic to brainstorm with students, as the classroom activity in Box 5.3 demonstrates. Recruitment is related to but distinct from sampling, as we discussed in the previous chapter.

You may choose to sample people who fit certain criteria, but you still also need to find those people, tell them about your study, and invite them to participate. An interview location may change depending on the nature of the project, but it almost always involves identifying somewhere safe and private, quiet, convenient (for the participant and the researcher), and comfortable—both physically and emotionally.

Box 5.3 Tips and tricks: Thinking through recruitment strategies and interview locations

---

Objective: helping students think through the logistics of recruitment. Where might you connect with people who have something to contribute to your study (i.e., information-rich participants)? How does recruitment shape the data you are likely to generate?

For this exercise, give your students several research scenarios with different target populations. Using the table below as a template, ask them to think through how they would recruit each population, possible challenges, and potential alternative recruitment strategies. In the table below, we provide a few research scenarios. You should pick your own with the goal of selecting scenarios that will best engage you and your students.

It can also be helpful for students to think through the process of selecting, logistics required for, ethical considerations of, and overall advantages and disadvantages of an interview location. The following table provides a structure to compare various considerations related to some typical locations for conducting research interviews. An in-class activity could be to provide students with one or two target populations (such as those in Table 5.1) with the instruction to consider each of the column headings for a specific group (see Table 5.2). For instance, if the population of interest is mothers with children under the age of 5, what would be the practical considerations of each possible location listed (the need for child care would be particularly critical)? How would rapport be likely impacted by each setting? Are there any ethical considerations (such as potentially witnessing familial interactions in the home that are outside of the scope of the study)? Will you possibly gain additional insight from the setting itself?

Table 5.1 Example matrix to help students consider practical aspects of recruitment for different types of participants

Target population	Recruitment venue	Method of recruitment	Possible limitations and barriers	Alternative recruitment strategies
Community health workers				
Out-of-care women living with HIV				
People with multiple sclerosis				
Mothers with children under the age of 5				

Table 5.2 Example matrix to help students consider the practical and conceptual dimensions of interview location

Interview location	Practical considerations	Rapport	Ethical considerations	Role of context
Office at the university				
Participant's home				
Cafe or library				
Someone's car				

Rapport

We spend considerable time discussing rapport, which we see as the ability to quickly create an interviewer-participant dynamic that is positive, relaxed, and mutually respectful. We often have our students brainstorm why building rapport with qualitative interview participants is so important. Generally, students can intuit that participants will talk more freely, openly, and honestly when they feel comfortable, trust the interviewer, feel secure about confidentiality, believe the interviewer is interested, and do not feel judged. Techniques for building rapport are somewhat culturally specific and topic dependent but often include being friendly, smiling, projecting relaxed body language, using a pleasant tone of voice, employing humor, demonstrating humility, practicing patience, and centering the participant's needs.

We teach our students how to use greetings and introductory statements before the official interview begins to help shape the participant's understanding of the interaction and what is expected of them. In the same sense, we use this discussion to demystify rapport-building. The interview itself may start with a broad explanation of the overall project, small talk or icebreaker questions, or some discussion of ground rules (e.g., that there are no right or wrong answers and that the participant can pause or end the interview at any time).

Consent

Until they have some experience with obtaining participants' consent, students may find this process somewhat mysterious and daunting. The core issue in the informed consent process is providing the potential participant with enough information about the study in the right circumstances to allow them to make an informed decision about whether they want to participate. Students may have many practical questions about the process—for example, whether they should read the consent form to the participant or let the participant read it. Practical details will vary by study and your institution, but you can explain some of the typical patterns of the process and the general principles that underpin decisions concerning consent in the context of qualitative research. The activity in Box 5.4. is one way to incorporate hands-on, real-world exploration of consent forms into the classroom.

Box 5.4 Tips and tricks: Introducing consent forms and consenting processes

As experienced researchers, we sometimes forget that students might not have exposure to or experience with the practicalities of informed consent, including consent forms and how and when to obtain consent. In our methods courses, we typically devote time to each of these issues. For the following exercise, you can use consent forms from your own research, your colleagues' projects, or examples from your institution's ethical review board. (The latter is especially useful if your institution has standardized templates.)

We recommend compiling a range of consent forms, such as the following:

- an oral consent form for a low-risk study, such as interviews with professionals about their jobs
- an oral consent form for a higher-risk study—for example, interviews in which patients or vulnerable populations will be asked about their personal experiences
- a written consent form for a qualitative study that requires longer engagement than a one-time interview or that will cover highly sensitive topics
- a written consent form for a clinical trial or similar study that includes extensive, detailed descriptions of study procedures, risks/harms, and protections (for comparison)

continued

Box 5.4 *continued*

This activity is intended to help students become familiar with the different types of consent forms they might use in research studies, compare the forms' format and content, and reflect on the process of obtaining consent and participant interaction.

After you've presented your students with an overview of the importance of informed consent in research and the ethical considerations of obtaining such consent, ask them to analyze and take notes on the similarities and differences in the consent forms. Instruct them to pay attention to the following aspects:

- **Format**: How is the information presented? Is it easy to understand?
- **Content**: What information does the consent form include? Does it outline the risks, benefits, and procedures of the study for the person who is considering participating?
- **Language**: Is the language jargon-free and comprehensible?
- **Consent process**: Are there sections that explain the voluntary nature of participation and the right to withdraw?

Then, either in groups or as a class, have your students share their observations. Invite them to share their insights and perspectives, drawing on their own experiences and observations. Encourage them to consider each form's strengths and weaknesses in terms of its clarity, accessibility, and effectiveness in conveying information. The discussion can focus on the following questions:

- How can different formats and styles of consent forms influence participants' comprehension and decision-making?
- What strategies can researchers employ to improve consent forms' clarity and effectiveness?
- How might participants' perceptions of the research study be influenced by its consent form?
- How can researchers ensure that their consent forms respect participants' autonomy and uphold ethical standards?

- How might the consent forms for qualitative and quantitative studies need to differ in their content, language, and approach?
- What might researchers consider when designing consent forms for different study types?
- How might participants' expectations and experiences vary between qualitative and quantitative research? How might this influence their interactions with consent forms?
- How can researchers ensure that their consent forms align with the specific ethical considerations of qualitative and quantitative research methodologies (Owczarzak & Smith, 2022)?

As a supplemental or complementary activity (possibly for a grade), you might have your students write a reflective essay on their understanding of the differences between qualitative and quantitative consent forms and how these differences reflect the unique ethical considerations of each research approach. Suggest that they consider examples from their field of study or personal experience.

Interview implementation

Then comes the meat (or plant-based protein ☺) of the interview—the actual data collection! Students will want to know what it's like to conduct an interview and how to do it well. At the most fundamental level, interview technique is about thinking and listening (Seidman, 2006): the interviewer asks questions, considers the participant's response, and uses it to shape the next question, as well as the course of the conversation. We talk about guiding the conversation so that the participant can share their perspective while the interviewer meets their goals. It takes time and practice to become a skilled qualitative interviewer; despite their enthusiasm, students won't be able to perfect the craft in a single course. We've been conducting interviews for decades and are still learning!

If you do not have the ability or resources for students to practice interviews within your course, you can still show them what a good qualitative interview should look like. Joanna Chrzanowska, a UK-based qualitative researcher, created demonstration videos to expose students to the basic mechanics and flow of a qualitative interview:

- *Qualitative interview with mistakes.*[1]
- *Demonstration qualitative interview: How it should be done.*[2]

Ask students to spot the mistakes (at least 10!) in the first video and then compare it to the second. You can use these videos to begin a class discussion of rapport-building, question-framing, probing, and how the different approaches influence the type of information the participant offers. Another way to expose students to the practical and real-world interview experience is through a panel of experts, as described in Box 5.5. Convening a panel of qualitative researchers with diverse data collection experiences (field site, data collection modality, prior training, etc.) to tell students about their experiences can help students develop a deeper understanding of the nuances of qualitative data collection.

There are also the logistical issues of recording and notetaking to consider. We review the goals of each: recording is best for capturing data during the interview, while notetaking allows the interviewer to listen and probe. We discuss the pros and cons of audio recording, video recording, and foregoing all recording in favor of written notes. Because of the difficulty of asking questions, listening to responses, and taking notes simultaneously, we advise students to always record their interviews, so long as it's possible to do so and participants agree. If the interviewer has built rapport and come to an agreement about how the data will be used, some form of recording will usually be possible.

Practical options for note formatting can be as simple as using blank paper or as involved as creating semi-structured forms that list

---

[1] Joanna Chrzanowska. (2014, July 9). *Qualitative interview with mistakes* [Video]. https://www.youtube.com/watch?v=U4UKwd0KExc.

[2] Joanna Chrzanowska. (2014, July 9). *Demonstration qualitative interview: How it should be done* [Video]. https://www.youtube.com/watch?v=eNMTJTnrTQQ.

key topics or questions and leave room for notes. When we cover this topic, we also talk about what can go wrong—not to scare students, but to prepare them for the technological and practical considerations of recording and notetaking. Planning for things to go wrong is well advised! We have had too many experiences of dead batteries on our recorders, thinking that we were recording when we weren't, or uploading a recording only to realize that the interviewee can barely be heard. In each case, it was critical to be able to pivot. Where can I buy batteries? Where can I charge or plug in my recording device? Can I create notes that can stand in for a recording that doesn't exist? Can I listen carefully to a bad audio file to capture as much detail as I can while my memory is still fresh? Do I need to attempt to reinterview the person? If I do this, how do I treat data that are somewhat reconstructed?

And of course, the work doesn't end when the interview does. We discuss different approaches to writing postinterview memos and team debriefing, along with transcription. We also like to address the different parts of an interview transcript and different transcription approaches, such as direct (i.e., word-for-word) transcription versus methods that seek only to capture the interview's essence. Furthermore, we talk about options for including nonverbal behavior, observations, and reactions in the transcript, and any additional details or data that might be helpful.

Box 5.5 Tips and tricks: Discussing practical aspects of data collection in diverse settings

Inviting a panel of qualitative experts to talk about their data collection experience can give students insights into the practical aspects of conducting interviews and undertaking other data collection in diverse settings. Researchers with experience in—to name a handful of examples—international settings, street-based recruitment, clinic recruitment, and

continued

Box 5.5 *continued*

the study of power dynamics (study up/study down) can provide students valuable knowledge about the challenges of and strategies involved with these contexts. A moderated panel may also allow you to focus on the practical aspects of interviewing and data collection in different settings.

Ask the panelists to share their experiences with and strategies for protocol development, training data collectors, obtaining consent, navigating power dynamics, and—of course—conducting interviews. Encourage the panelists to share challenges they've faced and lessons they've learned. This can be an informal exchange.

As a supplementary or complementary activity, ask students to write a short, reflective essay on one or more of the following topics, or have students discuss in small groups:

- What were their main takeaways from the panel discussion?
- How do practical considerations for interviews and data collection differ across settings?
- What strategies could researchers employ to address setting-specific challenges?
- How might cultural differences influence the interview process and data collection in international settings?
- Which ethical considerations are most important to keep in mind when conducting research with marginalized or vulnerable populations?
- How will the student apply this knowledge in their own research?

Individual and team-based approaches to conducting interviews

We like to talk about selecting and training interviewers. Some projects are run by a single researcher, responsible for all interviews and analysis. But public health research often involves working in teams, which means that students may have to decide who will conduct interviews and how to train those individuals. Students are often interested in whether interviewers and interviewees need to share sociodemographic or other characteristics. We use this topic to introduce the benefits and possible drawbacks of trying to match interviewers and participants in different studies and contexts. There are also cases when an interviewer may need to work with a translator or interpreter; decisions about selecting, training, and working with these members of the interview team can be critical for success.

An additional topic—one that may be more appropriate for advanced courses—is elite interviewing, also known as "interviewing up": interviewing people in power, such as community leaders, professionals, and policymakers. Techniques for elite interviewing may become a central skill for some students, one they will use and appreciate later in their careers.

Practicing interview skills

Given the very practical nature of teaching interviewing skills, you will almost certainly want students to at least observe an interview, if not practice conducting one themselves. If you haven't set up your course to allow for this, or if you want to employ the Socratic method, you can still demonstrate many of the above topics by bringing a student or TA to the front of the classroom with you and conducting a mock interview with them. You can then ask the class what they noticed about the interview: what went well, what didn't, and what the process can teach them about good interviewing techniques. You can also assign a video of one of your own qualitative interviews (if you have permission to do so), or one from another resource, including websites that curate qualitative interviews that were collected as part of a research project, as Box 5.6 suggests.

Box 5.6 Tips and tricks: Using online videos of qualitative interviews

---

To give students a realistic sense of the data generated by a qualitative interview, we have used the patient experience videos from the Health Experiences Research Network (HERN).[3] HERN was generated out of a research initiative of which two of this book's authors are a part—but the website interview video clips are a resource available to everyone. A limitation of these videos is their focus on the interview responses, rather than the work of the interviewer; regardless, the fact that they represent real qualitative data generated by a qualitative interview can be quite informative. Other interview examples (albeit not academic interviews) include digital audio archives of the Library of Congress and local historical societies. You can watch and discuss these during class or have your students watch on their own.

[3] Health Experiences Research Network. (n.d.). https://www.healthexperiencesusa.org/.

If one of your course's learning objectives is preparing students to conduct interviews, you'll want to have them practice conducting an interview at least once. You can arrange for this in several ways: your students can interview each other, they can interview someone they know, or they can interview someone from the community.

In summary, interviews are the most common form of data collection in qualitative public health research. For many of us, they are also often the most engaging and fun part of the work. It is a privilege to have people tell you about important experiences and to share their opinions and perspectives. It is also work that takes skill and practice to do well—and not everyone takes to the less structured style of qualitative interviewing easily.

Focus groups

As with interviews, we find that students are likely to join a qualitative methods course thinking they know at least a little about focus groups—and with the sense that focus groups are an essential qualitative method (if not *the* essential method). We have also found that students often have misconceptions about what a focus group is, when to use one, and the data generated. We therefore recommend starting your discussion of focus groups by engaging with the basics: what a focus group is, what it is not, when it might be useful, and when it would likely not generate useful data. Box 5.7 highlights some of the primary differences between interviews and focus groups in terms of the practicalities of implementation and the type of data they generate.

At its core, a focus group is a process of bringing people together to talk with each other about a research topic relevant to them. Focus groups are conversations that are facilitated or moderated by the researcher or someone else with specific training. As with an individual interview, the structure of focus groups can take many forms, with a preference for questions that are open-ended (Schensul & LeCompte, 2012). Because focus groups are comprised of multiple participants, interaction around a topic of interest by people with some shared characteristic is a key component of this method. Frequently, focus groups are used to understand how group members talk with each other about a given topic; they can provide insights into within-group language and norms. Similarly, because a focus group's process of "sharing and comparing" (Morgan, 1997) may facilitate deeper insights into a given topic, its participants are encouraged to talk to each other, with limited guidance from the facilitator.

A focus group produces a distinct form of data; it is not a way for the researcher to get the same information from multiple people in a single session, nor are focus groups a more efficient data collection process than individual interviews. Box 5.8 presents an overview of some of the common myths and realities of conducting focus groups that you may need to debunk in a methods class.

As we emphasize throughout this book, the research question should shape methods choices. Too often, we encounter both seasoned researchers and novice students who propose focus groups because they think that they will be "quick." The assumption is that focus groups are valuable because this will allow the researcher to talk to a lot of people at once. Our experience collecting qualitative data shows us that the decision to conduct focus groups should not be one of expediency (which is often a false assumption). It is important that the decision be intentional and in response to a specific research need.

Given that multiple people will contribute their experience and perspective to the topic in a single session, focus groups work better when the researcher can take a minimalist approach to topics and questions posed. The goal is to facilitate conversations between group participants, and also to allow for full participation by all. The skills required for an effective focus group facilitator are distinct from those needed for a rich qualitative interview; a focus group facilitator is tasked with establishing and maintaining good group dynamics whereas a qualitative interviewer is seeking one-on-one connection and trust.

A focus group facilitator (whether this be the researcher or a professional hired to take this on) shouldn't expect to bring the same interview guide, with its long list of topics and questions, and cover the same amount of territory with a focus group as one might in an interview. It is much more likely that a focus group facilitator who is well trained and oriented to the research question(s) will have success with a more limited set of interview domains and varied possible discussion prompts.

It is important for researchers to be thoughtful about topics for a focus group. Highly personal experiences with sensitive, stigmatized topics (e.g., substance use, mental health, exposure to violence) may be inappropriate for a group discussion. Helping students understand the strengths, limitations, and caveats of focus groups can, in turn, help them make informed decisions about the most appropriate method of data collection for their goals.

Box 5.7 Tips and tricks: Comparing interviews and focus groups

---

As a class exercise, have your students pair up and give them 10 minutes to generate a list of the pros and cons of qualitative interviews and focus groups, and to brainstorm ideas for sample questions that align well with each. Then, have them defend their ideas to the class. They may come up with a table like the one below in Table 5.3.

Table 5.3 Example table to compare pros and cons of interviews and focus groups

	Interviews	Focus groups
Strengths	- individual stories and experiences - privacy and confidentiality - increases likelihood that data collected are on topic-concentrates insight on cognitive thoughts and decision-making processes - examines phenomena that are inherently unobservable because they are rare, unpredictable, or private (earthquakes, sex)	- good sense of social norms, how participants talk with each other about a topic - direct evidence of similarities and differences across individual experiences - safety in numbers - capacity to generate insights based on others' experiences
Limitations	- what people say they do rather than what they do	- participants frame their responses for the researchers and for each other (i.e., possible social desirability bias) - lack of privacy - limited time for each person

---

Box 5.8 Tips and tricks: Debunking common misperceptions about focus groups

To help students understand what focus groups are and how to use them most effectively, you may need to debunk some of the ideas they bring to the classroom. Below, in Table 5.4, are some of the inaccurate assumptions about focus groups we've encountered in the classroom and suggestions for how to reshape your students' understanding of them.

Table 5.4 Breaking down myths about focus groups

Myth	Fact
Focus groups are the primary method of qualitative data collection.	Focus groups are one method out of many. The data collection method should fit the research question.
Conducting one focus group with 10 participants is essentially the same thing as conducting 10 interviews.	The group is the unit of analysis, not the number of participants. The interplay between both individual and group levels of analysis contributes to the data. The type of information collected through a focus group is therefore different from the type collected through interviews.
Focus groups are an easy way of gathering a lot of qualitative data relatively quickly.	Good focus groups take a lot of logistical planning and require a skilled facilitator. Data collection is unlikely to be quick or easy, and data analysis definitely won't be!

As with teaching individual interviews, you decide how much course content you want to devote to the history, purpose, and practicalities of conducting focus groups. Courses more aligned with an appreciation of the methods may focus on how focus groups were popularized in the 1950s as a market research tool for understanding consumer behavior, preferences, and motivations, as well as the reasons for choosing them over other methods. In other words, such a course would prioritize the pros and cons of focus groups. And while focus groups do remain an important market research tool—for example, to obtain feedback on new products—the method has also been widely adapted by the social sciences, including public health. Focus groups can be used to learn about group attitudes and how participants interact with each other, resulting in different insights than those that occur when participants are engaging one-on-one with an interviewer.

To help students appreciate the utility of focus groups, you might identify a peer-reviewed article that used focus groups and have students evaluate how the author operationalized focus groups to answer their research question, how they structured the focus groups (e.g., the number of participants in each group, the number of groups, group composition, group size), and the analytical insights or findings the method produced. Then, have students brainstorm how the data and findings would look different if the same research question had been explored through individual interviews instead of groups.

For classes on skill-building and research design, discussion of focus groups could also include practical considerations for structuring focus groups, such as the following:

- the number and size of groups
- group composition: whom to match with whom (both participants and moderators)
- specific ethical concerns with group-based methods
- greetings, ground rules, icebreaker questions, and closing statements

Box 5.9 offers one structured activity to help students think through the logistics of planning and conducting a focus group.

Box 5.9 Tips and tricks: Planning a focus group

Another classroom activity that can also work well as a take-home assignment is to present students with a scenario in which they will conduct a focus group, including a research question and a description of the population. Have your students write a plan for organizing the focus group that includes a justification for the organizational decisions they make.

The following are three examples that we have used:

- a study on substance use after incarceration that seeks to include the perspectives of people who were formally incarcerated, correctional officers, community supervision professionals, and family members of those who've been incarcerated
- a study of the experience of cancer treatment that seeks to include the perspectives of people undergoing treatment, family and friends who provide informal care for those undergoing treatment, and oncology professionals
- a study of how a gun-violence prevention policy is being implemented at the local level from the perspective of community members impacted by violence, including youth, veterans, and people who survived suicide

You might ask students to address some of the following questions:

Overview

- Are focus groups appropriate for the topic and population of interest?

Setting up the focus group

- Who will be responsible for focus group logistics—who will serve as facilitator, notetaker, and coordinate on-site or online details? What skills or background should people in these roles have?

- How will you recruit participants?
- How will you organize the groups? By age, by gender, by role? How many people need to be in each group? Justify your organizational structure.
- Will you compensate participants? If so, how, and how much?
- Where will you hold the focus group? How will you accommodate participants' needs (e.g., child care)?

Conducting the focus group

- What skills does your facilitator need? How will you identify or develop these skills?
- What group rules might you need to establish?
- What kind of activities, stimulus, or other media will you incorporate into the discussion? Why these materials? How will you use them?
- What kinds of questions are appropriate to ask in the focus group?
- How will you ensure you get quality data that cover the full range of issues, have appropriate depth and specificity, and facilitate both personal context and the process of sharing and comparing across participants?

Managing focus group data

- How will you use the discussion notes?
- Who will transcribe the audio recordings? How will you keep track of each speaker within the transcribed text?

Because online focus groups are increasingly common, you can also incorporate a discussion of the pros, cons, and practical considerations of such groups into your consideration of focus groups. This discussion might include student reflections on their own experiences using online platforms for classes and other activities. Encourage students to describe what they think works well, what the challenges are, and what they would do to improve the experience—including how to get people to participate.

A focus group's practical aspects may be difficult to practice or replicate in the classroom, but giving students a protocol or planning document will help them appreciate the logistical considerations to account for when undertaking a focus group (see Box 5.10). Unlike individual interviews, focus groups require more than the typical consent form and audio recorder: food, a focus group guide, a notetaker, space to accommodate the group, and considerations for child care are all common when hosting a focus group. Focus groups may also use media, such as intervention elements or advertisements, to which participants will be asked to react and which require additional planning to execute (see Box 5.11). Focus groups might require the facilitator to keep track of comments on a whiteboard or flipchart and help other participants know what to respond to. Showing students a checklist of materials and a general agenda for a focus group, as in Box 5.10, can help them appreciate considerations for success.

Box 5.10 Qualitative building blocks: What you need on the day of the focus group

---

Materials

- consent forms
- pens
- audio recorders and microphones (specific to recording groups)
- media or other interactive materials
- flipchart
- markers
- snacks or a meal, depending on the time of day

- incentives
- facilitation guides

Procedures

- check-in and logistics
- consent process
- overview and group purpose
- nature of participation
- establishing ground rules (confidentiality, turn-taking)
- participant introductions
- main discussion
- thank you and conclusion

Practicing focus group skills

As with interviews, the best ways to learn how to run a focus group are observing how experienced facilitators run them and experiencing facilitating them yourself. Hands-on experience can be a class exercise—either with students or with people from outside the class. However, you have to consider the time you have available in the course: a focus group's logistics are more daunting than those of an individual interview. These logistics may also make it difficult for each student to practice each focus group role: facilitator, notetaker, and logistics coordinator.

A classroom setting can offer an opportunity for students to observe a mock focus group.

Another option is showing and having your students evaluate a video of a focus group previously conducted for this purpose. We would advise that in either case the focus group should be as realistic as possible with an experienced facilitator, a group of participants with a genuine interest in common (it would be important to identify an issue with high engagement but low emotion, perhaps something like avoiding injury while training for a competitive sport), to have a discussion for about 20 minutes. Students observing can be prompted to give consideration to issues such as the following:

- Were all participants equally engaged or represented in the discussion?
- Did the conversation flow between participants or bounce back and forth to the facilitator?
- Were there issues raised by a participant that were not followed up on because the conversation went in a different direction?
- How much agreement or disagreement emerged from the discussion?

It may also be insightful to have the group participants debrief on their experience in the group, as the think-pair-share activity in Box 5.11 presents. Did they feel that they were able to fully participate? Were there experiences/opinions that they would have shared one-on-one but didn't feel comfortable sharing in the group? Were there some issues that were raised by others that they wouldn't have thought to raise but were pertinent to them?

Box 5.11 Tips and tricks: Evaluating a focus group

You can use the think-pair-share approach following a classroom demonstration of a professor-led focus group. Open-ended questions may include, "Where were areas of agreement and disagreement among participants?" "Which techniques did the moderator use to generate discussion?" "What could the moderator have done to draw out quieter participants or ensure that the conversation remained on topic?" You may even create a list of ideas, then add any additional skills you want to make sure your students learn.

Observations

Observational research is a process whereby events, behaviors (including conversations and interpersonal interactions), and social objects are studied systematically, within a social context beyond the parameters of research (Marshall & Rossman, 1989). Learning about a topic or issue firsthand is at the heart of classic qualitative methodology; observational methods are often considered the gold standard for research that intends to understand a phenomenon by considering what people do, in addition to how they might describe or explain it (Green & Thorogood, 2004). Observational research exemplifies a form of real-world data collection in which complexity is embraced, rather than controlled. For all of these reasons, you may choose to start your introduction of the major data collection approaches with observation. It is also possibly more straightforward to provide students with some experience in conducting this type of research. On the other hand, students are less likely to come to the course anticipating this type of research approach—and having exposure to talk-based methods (interviews and focus groups) can help students to grasp the specific contributions of observational methods.

Unlike with interviews and focus groups, most students who join our courses have little sense of what observational research is, why it's valuable, and how they might go about conducting it. By the end of our courses, we strive to have demonstrated why sometimes the best data come from watching and being a part of social life—not just asking people about it. Box 5.12 uses the example of Max Weber's theory of social action and chopping wood to illustrate how different types and levels of engagement among the researcher, the participant, and the phenomenon of interest can reveal different dimensions of a social experience.

Box 5.12 Tips and tricks: Revisiting the connection between methods and questions

Max Weber's theory of social action references differences between what a person/researcher can learn by observing a man chopping wood and by asking him about his experience chopping wood. To introduce students to this idea, we find that an illustration of someone chopping wood is an excellent prop for a class discussion on the different questions that might be appropriate for observational methods in comparison with interviewing.

We display such an illustration at the beginning of class and ask our students to imagine observing this person for 15–20 minutes. What kinds of questions could they answer with the data from their observations? Their responses tend to include the following:

- What type of ax does the woodchopper use?
- What is their swing like?
- Does the woodchopper take breaks?
- How big are the pieces they cut?
- Does the woodchopper do this alone, or with other people?

All of these questions can be answered—at least partially—by observing. In addition, the following are some of the questions that students often also suggest and that we ask them to think about further, *as they would be better answered by talking with the person engaged in the activity than by observation alone*:

- Why is this person chopping wood?
- How do they select what wood to chop?
- Is chopping wood pleasurable or painful?

Finally, we ask students to imagine spending 10 minutes engaging in the activity (participant observation). Figure 5.3 illustrates the question of what they could learn by doing the activity or combining the various data collection approaches.

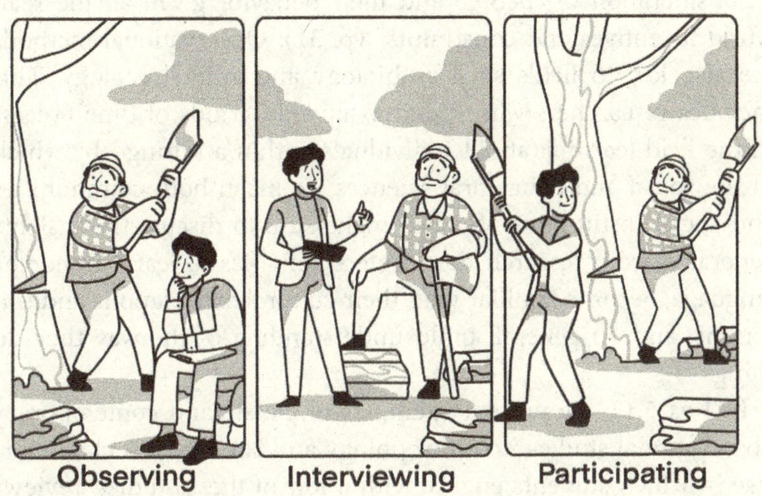

Figure 5.3 Illustration of observing, interviewing, and participating to learn about woodchopping

Even though students are often less familiar with observational research, we always spend time introducing this approach in our qualitative public health courses. It is a foundational method to qualitative research; data collected through observation are not easily obtained through other approaches. We believe that it is also an underappreciated method in public health. Alumni from our courses can serve as ambassadors and advocates for the value of ethnography and participant observation in meeting public health objectives.

What data are generated through observational research?

Discussions of the value of observational research for addressing public health concerns can be anchored in the long, rich history of ethnography in fields such as anthropology and sociology. Fetterman (1998) has described ethnography as facilitating a consideration of "people and their behavior given all the real-world incentives and constraints" (p. 31). Observational methods are also key to fields such as biology and animal ecology. This includes researchers who spend extended periods of time (years) in the field learning about individuals within a setting—by which in the social and behavioral sciences we mean both communities and social institutions. We also make sure to discuss the insights generated from research that centers activities to learn a people's language, become familiar with their cultural expectations and traditions, and, in general, build understanding of the way they do things.

In Box 5.13, we present examples of classic and contemporary observational studies in anthropology and sociology. A class exercise in which students engage with a few of these studies' reviews can help illustrate the kinds of questions that these methods can help answer.

Box 5.13 Qualitative building blocks: Examples of ethnographic and observational studies from anthropology and sociology

---

- Biruk, C. (2018). *Cooking data: Culture and politics in an African research world*. Duke University Press.
- Bosk, C. (2003). *Forgive and remember: Managing medical failure*. University of Chicago Press.
- Closser, S. (2010). *Chasing polio in Pakistan: Why the world's largest public health initiative may fail*. Vanderbilt University Press.
- Fadiman, A. (2012). *The spirit catches you and you fall down: A Hmong child, her American doctors, and the collision of two cultures*. Macmillan.
- Glaser, B. G., & Strauss, A. L. (1965). *Awareness of dying*. Aldine.

- Qureshi, K. (2019). *Chronic illness in a Pakistani labour diaspora*. Carolina Academic Press.
- Solimeo, S. (2009). *With shaking hands: Aging with Parkinson's disease in America's heartland*. Rutgers University Press.

Accessing the setting

Before observing anything, the researcher needs access to a research setting. Prompt your students to think in practical terms about where they might conduct observations for a given research question.

- Do they know where the action they want to observe happens?
- Would they belong in the setting if they weren't there for research?
- Would they have to ask permission to be in the setting if they weren't conducting research? (For example, is the space public or private?)
- Is it clear who has the right to grant access to the setting?

The process of gaining access to a research setting can be formal or informal, but research ethics include the general expectation that the researcher will inform others in the setting where observation is taking place, as well as the nature of the observation. Access, even if informal, is part of ensuring such awareness. For more on research ethics, see Chapter 7.

We push students who are in courses to prepare them to lead their own research to consider these ethical issues more thoroughly. For instance, we show a photograph of a city park and ask students whether they need permission to conduct observational research in a public place such as this. Our follow-up questions include the following:

- Do any of the following variables matter—and, if so, to what extent?
    - the identity of the observer
    - the identity of the observed
    - the duration of the observation
    - what the observed are doing
    - the distance between observer and observed
    - the observer's recording method
- To the extent that permission is necessary, how does the researcher get permission?

All of these questions are intended to facilitate students giving careful consideration to the possible risks and/or ethical challenges of research in a setting that at first may seem innocuous or low risk. This exercise doesn't come with a set of strictly correct answers—there aren't ones to give. But it does put aside the notion that public observation is simple. To be sure, there are some general principles—private spaces, such as a home, usually require full consent; semipublic spaces, such as a clinic waiting room, usually require consent from gatekeepers at a minimum; and fully public spaces may require consent only for specific situations. But ethical considerations of observational access and consent are complex enough that even IRB members often discuss (and differ on!) how to handle some of these gray areas.

Gold's typology of observational methods

A common distinction in the conduct of observational research is between the emic perspective—that of an insider—and the etic, or outsider, perspective. Students may gravitate toward the idea that insiders are better observers. Fetterman (1998) has argued that some level of distance is key, stating that "[p]articipant observation combines participation in the lives of the people under study with the maintenance of a professional distance that allows adequate observation and recording of data" (p. 35). In our courses, we emphasize that neither position is necessarily "better" but rather that people coming from emic or etic perspectives will likely take note of different things in a given setting, and thus these approaches are not interchangeable but rather complementary.

Gold's (1958) typology presented four potential roles for a researcher in an observational study: complete participant, participant-as-observer, observer-as-participant, and complete observer. A class discussion of this typology can help students consider the observer's differential impact on a setting based on what they're doing in the setting and the extent to which they belong there. Table 5.5 provides some examples of the different ways that levels of immersion can be applied to different research questions and settings. Students should also be prompted to think about the effect of the observer's familiarity with and comfort in the setting on the data they generate. Box 5.14 describes one classroom activity to help students reflect on both the practicalities and epistemological dimensions of observational research.

Table 5.5 Application of Gold's typology of observer roles

Role type	Role description	Example applications
Complete participant	The researcher's role in the setting beyond their research does not change during the research. It is possible that only they know their identity as a researcher. Complete observer is not, however, synonymous with covert observer.	Researcher receives health care services and draws on that experience to inform their observation. A pregnant researcher goes to pregnancy yoga classes and later "mommy and me" events to learn about gender and motherhood.
	In addition, the researcher can use their own experiences—not intended for research—as data.	Researcher is a health educator in a school system and receives training on suicide prevention. She then applies this in her work and studies the impact on her students' engagement with this topic.

continued

Table 5.5 *continued*

Role type	Role description	Example applications
Participant-as-observer	The researcher has an ongoing role in the setting. Anyone in the setting can be aware of the primacy (or not) of the research in interactions. There are times when the researcher will be in the setting explicitly for research purposes.	Researcher is a nurse whose research is seeking to understand sources of discrimination in medicine through his clinical role. A member of a research team engaged in intervention research also conducts an ethnography of the research itself. Researcher provides technical assistance to a state health department team charged with implementing regulations for overdose prevention sites. The research team is evaluating uptake of the overdose prevention sites by people who use drugs.
Observer-as-participant	The researcher enters the setting for their study and has a role beyond that of observer. (Often, this role develops over time.) Everyone in the setting understands that the researcher's role in the setting is limited primarily to the research.	Researcher embeds in a local public health department as part of an ethnography and takes on limited tasks over time. Researcher trains local health department staff on a new child-passenger safety policy and observes child-passenger safety services provided by the staff in the community.
Complete observer	The researcher enters the setting for the study's purposes and has no role there other than to observe. Furthermore, the researcher is positioned such that the participants do not need to take the researcher into account, and may not even know that they are being observed.	Researcher observes blood pressure check intervention delivered at a community health fair. Researcher accompanies a community health worker on their daily home visits but doesn't interact with clients or provide services. Researcher observes public hearings on a gun violence prevention bill held by a state legislative committee.

Box 5.14 Tips and tricks: Demonstrating the observer's positionality

Because observation is part of everyday life, it can be difficult to envision the challenges of conducting research by placing oneself in a social setting to monitor and record either most or a specific element of what happens there. It can therefore be useful for students to imagine the effect on the research of their comfort level, or the extent to which they are accepted in a setting. This is not to say that the best observational research is done by people who feel comfortable and accepted—only that these elements shape the experience.

To help your students imagine this, have them place themselves in two or three distinct social settings—spots where they feel like they belong, or feel either comfortable or not comfortable—for around 10 minutes each. Have them take notes not on what they observe, but on their feelings and the things that they are aware of that they do and don't have access to in the setting. After their observations, have your students reflect upon their notes in small groups and present the themes that emerge to the full class. You may also want to ask them to consider how they chose their settings and how their choices did or did not serve them well. Did people seem to notice them? Do they think that their observing caused people to change their behavior?

Observational structure; frameworks for observation

In learning about observation, students must first understand why they might observe in the first place. They can then become keen observers of their surroundings, recognizing what is important in a given setting and documenting their observations in careful field notes.

A good observational exercise (as a part of class or as homework) has your students once again placing themselves in a public setting for a 10-minute observation. (This time, students can observe in pairs, if they like.) Settings might include the following:

- a park bench
- a bus stop, train station, or airport waiting lounge
- a campus coffee shop or cafeteria
- outside a busy grocery store
- a shopping mall
- a sporting event
- on public transportation (this setting can double as a way for students to get to know a new community!)

While observing, students are to take field notes using one or two of Creswell's (2016) prompts:

- Write a chronology of events that occur during the observation.
- Describe what you experience using at least four of the senses.
- Before you observe, write down two or three questions that ask what you want to learn; then, record by trying to answer them.
- Draw a picture or diagram of the setting.
- Write a narrative of the observational time.
- The setting may make it possible to collect two sets of data—one in which the student only observes (pure observation) and another in which they are engaged in the setting's activity (participant observation). What's notable about each experience?
- Reflect on the challenges experienced and problems faced during the observation and the questions raised by conducting the observation.

Following the observation, have your students spend up to 15 minutes in a separate location to continue addressing their chosen prompts. They should then spend five minutes writing about what they could record in the setting, what they could only record after leaving it, and how both types of field notes might serve as research data. Students who work in pairs can compare their notes and data and consider what may have led to any differences.

In your class, you may wish to explicitly help students to differentiate "descriptive notes"—that is, notes on what happened in the setting—and "reflexive notes," or notes on how what happened made you think about or feel, in any observational activity (Creswell, 2016). It may also be helpful to provide your students with suggestions for structuring their field notes: they might break them down into two separate journals or integrate them into a single narrative, split down the left and right sides of a page.

For online or hybrid courses, a video can be a tool to give the class a shared observational experience. We've had considerable success mimicking the in-person exercise above by playing a news story of a gun show. The clip we use is just over two minutes and features a walk-through of a typical gun show in the United States, including brief interviews with gun sellers and parents who brought their children. We've also used a news clip of a New York City restaurant's adaptations to COVID-19. The clips encourage students to imagine these social worlds and the public-health-related research questions each setting would allow them to explore.

Documents and artifacts

Students may not have considered the amount they can learn about the social world through a detailed and systematic examination of items, artifacts, and documents that exist in the social world apart from the research realm. Miller (1997, p. 2) has described social texts as an important facet of how we "construct, sustain, contest and change our senses of social reality." There are a vast array of objects pertinent to public health; a few examples of public health objects are items such as COVID-19 test kits (or even an object such as a mask), CDC growth charts, a medical school curriculum on a given medical condition, a cigarette pack, a magazine ad for vodka, a TV ad for a weight loss drug, a city ordinance related to air pollution.

A constructivist approach to learning from social objects (see Chapter 3) is sometimes called "discourse analysis." In such an approach, the focus is on the ways that important social elements are produced, reproduced, and changed (Green & Thorogood, 2004).

Among the most essential issues related to teaching qualitative research of documents or social artifacts are the following:

- the kinds of research questions answerable by an analysis of artifacts/documents
- the artifacts/documents to be included in the research (sampling)
- how to engage with the artifacts systematically (analysis)
- what documents and social artifact can or cannot tell us

Example research questions addressed by document analysis include the following:

- Which workplace policies are related to sick leave? How is illness described in such policies (e.g., is mental health explicitly included? Is caregiving for family members included?)
- How have ideas about infectious disease changed since the COVID-19 pandemic as demonstrated through news coverage of outbreaks?
- How is climate change's influence on health being discussed on social media—over time, between countries, within different populations?

One of the first tasks in teaching the use of documents as qualitative research data is getting students to think about the *kinds* of documents and social artifacts there are in the world and how students might use them to improve their own understanding of a social phenomenon. As Box 5.15 illustrates, there are many different types of objects that can be part of a document analysis! Increasingly, these will be digital artifacts, which can pose some important methodological questions.

Box 5.15 Tips and tricks: What types of objects can be usefully analyzed to address public health questions?

Your students may appreciate specific examples of the kinds of objects that could be beneficial for a document or artifact analysis. Here is a brief list of documents that we have used in our research that we sometimes reference in our classes. This list is not intended to be exhaustive.

- news articles
- public records
- letters and diaries
- organizational products
- reports and presentations
- legal and policy documents (e.g., hearing testimony, legislative bills, public comment in the rulemaking process)
- social media posts
- photographs and other images
- research products (e.g., journal articles)
- videos
- speeches
- websites
- public service announcements and campaigns
- meeting notes and agendas
- products (e.g., cigarette packs, medicine packaging)

Artifacts—including documents—are valuable as research data because they are the products of social acts and reflect the temporal and cultural contexts that produced them. Their research purpose will depend on the research question and the researcher's perspective (Green & Thorogood, 2004). To get your students thinking in these terms, you might pose a broad research question or a series of questions and have the class discuss the relevant documents or artifacts that might be available, as well as what gathering and analyzing such data would yield compared with other methods. Another useful exercise could be to have your students generate their own research questions for examination with document analysis and have them debate, in small groups, the pros and cons of using documents as data in each case.

Topics to consider when teaching the use of documents and social artifacts as data

- Why might you include documents or artifacts in your research?
- How can you identify documents or artifacts relevant to your research question? (i.e., what is the nature of your source material?)
- How would you construct an analytic sample?
    - What are the types of documents?
    - What is the relevant time period to define your document search?
    - Will you analyze every available document, or sample?
- What questions will you ask of the data?

Altheide (2000) has called qualitative document analysis "similar to all qualitative methodology in that the main emphasis is on discovery and description, including search[ing] for underlying meanings, patterns and processes, rather than mere quantity or numerical relationships between two or more variables" (p. 290). Processes of analyzing or making meaning from documents include "finding, selecting, appraising (making sense of) and synthesizing data contained in documents" (Bowen, 2009, p. 28). Box 5.16 provides a classroom activity or homework assignment that can help students think holistically and contextually about objects as part of a social world to be examined and understood.

How can documents or artifacts be used as data?

- Documents can provide data on the context in which people operate (Bowen, 2009).
- Documents can be used to track change (Bowen, 2009).
- Documents can help explain otherwise unavailable perspectives (e.g., it may be possible to learn about a person unable or unwilling to be interviewed through that person's writings).
- Documents are not interchangeable with other forms of qualitative research data (e.g., what someone tells a researcher in an interview or what a researcher might observe them doing).
- Documents can allow for the triangulation of data generated via other methods.

Box 5.16 Tips and tricks: Analyzing artifacts

A class that teaches artifact analysis can contextualize the study of objects within the broader framing of the social world as replete with things: those that people use and make in everyday life, that embody and express social relationships, that express our tastes and reflect our social status and position, and that convey special meaning or significance. To do this with an assignment that combines take-home work and in-class discussion, try a guided artifact analysis. Have your students identify a material object that they understand people consider to be meaningful or that sums up or otherwise expresses a system of value or meaning (e.g., an American flag). After they bring to class either a picture of the object or the object itself,

continued

Box 5.16 *continued*

---

your students can use the following set of questions to delve deeper into the object's significance.

Evoke an image: Write a physical description of the object
Describe the object's physical attributes, including the following:

- material
- color, size, shape, and weight
- markings or symbols
- condition/quality
- what the artifact shows
- what is absent from the artifact

If your object contains images and text, discuss the following questions:

- What was the creator of the item's purpose in and context for making it?
    - original historical, cultural, social, political context
- What does the item depict? How is it represented?
    - identity, character, personality, status, symbolism
    - the story behind the item's creation (e.g., decode the social/cultural context)
    - what is included
    - what is excluded
- What is the relationship between text and other elements of the item?
- Which ideas, concepts, and/or emotions are conveyed?

FOLLOW THE OBJECT: Illuminate the object's biography, including how its use and meaning change by time and context
Describe the ways the object is used in your field setting.

- What is the object's purpose?

- Who uses it?
  - Who is the intended user (an individual or a group)?
  - Who cannot or does not use it?
  - Do different people use it differently?
- How public is the object?
- Which social relationships and roles does the object create or maintain?
- How is the object similar to and different from others in the same category?

Place the object into a broader social and historical context.

- What background information makes this object intelligible to others?
- What happened—in society, in history—when this object was made?
- If someone within the setting made the object:
  - Who made it?
  - How did they make it?
  - What skills, tools, and training were required to make it?
- If the object was created elsewhere, how did this person or this group acquire it?

DETERMINE THE MEANING: Explore how this object is a vehicle for cultural meaning and the meaning that it communicates

Think about your object's symbolic dimensions.

- What is the object's meaning for its users?
- Has its meaning or use changed over time?
- Is its meaning different for different users?
- What message does it communicate?

SUMMARIZE YOUR OBJECT: Describe the cultural significance of your object

continued

Box 5.16 *continued*

Write a paragraph describing what your object can tell us about the following aspects of your field site:

- traditions
- rituals
- values
- rules
- behaviors

In Chapter 6, we will turn to teaching qualitative analysis. For document and artifact research, there is not the same data construction work as with interviews, focus groups, and observations. It is more challenging to differentiate data construction and analysis in document analysis.

Altheide (2000) has outlined the following steps for qualitative document analysis:

1. Identify the problem to be investigated.
2. Explore the possible sources of existing information (i.e., documents or artifacts).
3. Become familiar with several relevant documents.
4. Select the unit of analysis (e.g., a news outlet, publication, or article).
5. List several categories to guide data collection sample construction.
6. Draft a coding guide or protocol.
7. Test and refine—possibly over many iterations—protocol using several diverse documents (pp. 291–292).

Bowen (2009) has outlined three steps for qualitative document analysis: skimming, reading, and interpretation. This process allows for identifying meaningful and relevant passages of text, followed by subjecting the emergent themes to a focused review of the data for analytic purposes. And, as with other analytic methods (see Chapter 5), the researcher can apply both predefined and emergent codes.

In the READ approach (Dalglish et al., 2021), a similar set of steps is followed:

1. Ready your materials.
2. Extract your data.
3. Analyze your data.
4. Distill your findings.

Document analysis is one area where it's relatively easy to prepare data sets for students to use in class exercises and gain firsthand experience. The method also lends itself to student construction of a purposive sample with authentic data related to an issue pertinent to them. Public records are a particularly good source of authentic research data; try asking your students to scan such records for documents that could be collected in response to a particular prompt and create an annotated list of the document name, type (e.g., report, advertisement), source (e.g., federal regulatory agency, media company), and information gleaned from analyzing it. One example is an annotated list of documents that demonstrate changing attitudes about and policies regarding tobacco: it could include FDA policy documents, cigarette marketing, indoor smoking policies, and media debates over electronic cigarettes. Box 5.17 provides a structured set of questions that can be incorporated into an assignment or in-class activity around document analysis.

Box 5.17 Tips and tricks: Practicing policy analysis

Bacchi's "What's the problem represented to be?" approach to policy analysis

Give your students either a policy document or a policy summary and have them review with the following questions in mind:

continued

Box 5.17 *continued*

---

1. What's the problem as represented by a specific policy?
2. What suppositions or assumptions underlie the representation of this problem?
3. How has this representation of the problem come about?
4. What does this representation leave unproblematic? Where are the silences? Can the problem be thought about differently?
5. What effects does this representation produce?
6. How and where has this representation been produced, disseminated, and defended?
7. How can the representation be questioned, disrupted, and replaced? (Bacchi, 2009, p. 2)

After completing this task, you can have your students apply this list to problem representations in areas of interest to them.

Social media analysis

A specific type of document analysis increasingly common in public health is social media analysis. Students are likely quite familiar with social media; many love the idea of analyzing these platforms for cultural trends and perspectives on health-related topics. Social media can be a good teaching tool to engage students in the idea and practicalities of conducting document analysis. Class exercises can focus on posts, as well as interactions with posts (both textual interaction and platform-generated interaction), user profiles, friend or social networks, hashtags, or advertising.

Summary

Interviews, focus groups, observations, and documents and artifacts can all provide valuable qualitative data. Teaching them can be fun and creative. Students need to know about the huge range of potential methods they can draw from—and what they might be able to learn from each one.

Additional readings on qualitative research methods

The following is a list of resources that you and/or your students may find to be particularly useful as grounding for aspects of the methods outlined in Chapter 5.

- Bowen, G. (2009). Document analysis as a qualitative research method. *Qualitative Research Journal*, 9(2), 27–40.
- Emerson, R. M., Fretz, R. I., & Shaw, L. L. (2011). *Writing ethnographic fieldnotes*. University of Chicago Press.
- Hammersley, M., & Atkinson, P. (2019). *Ethnography: Principles in practice*. Routledge.
- Hennink, M. M., Kaiser, B. N., & Weber, M. B. (2019). What influences saturation? Estimating sample sizes in focus group research. *Qualitative Health Research, 29*(10), 1483–1496.
- Morgan, D. (1997). *Focus groups as qualitative research* (2nd ed.). Sage Publications.
- Patton, M. Q. (2002). *Qualitative research & evaluation methods* (3rd ed.). Sage Publications.
- Spradley, J. P. (2016). *The ethnographic interview*. Waveland Press.

6

Teaching qualitative analysis and how to write up qualitative research

Introduction

Qualitative analysis is, according to C. Wright Mills, a form of "intellectual craftmanship" (Mills, 1959, p. 195). It is also often the most challenging and the most rewarding part of the research process. Because this step involves craft, it can be difficult to develop and teach. Our approach to teaching qualitative analysis is informed by the recognition that keeping students engaged with and confident in their own abilities requires us to apply extra effort to the analysis itself. We intend Chapter 6 to describe this approach: we explain the tools and principles we use to make meaning from qualitative—usually textual—data.

The nature of your course should be responsive to your students' prior exposure to qualitative data. Some students may have experience collecting data themselves; others may have no hands-on exposure to qualitative data and all they know is what they've learned from you. Accounting for this range is important for knowing where to begin when teaching analysis. In our experience, it's common for students to have no prior exposure to a complete interview transcript or a complete data set with many transcripts before they join our courses. You will need to adapt the instructional techniques in relation to your students' prior exposure to qualitative data and learning

Teaching Qualitative Research in Public Health. Katherine Clegg Smith et al., Oxford University Press.
© Oxford University Press (2026). DOI: 10.1093/9780197662472.003.0006

objectives. If you are teaching a stand-alone qualitative methods course, as we do, considering prerequisites and what expectations you will have for students on Day 1, and what you are willing to teach to ensure everyone is ready to dig into analysis, are important considerations.

Here, qualitative data analysis refers to three distinct, interrelated processes: **coding**, **analysis**, and **interpretation**.

When we code data, we organize it; we summarize, synthesize, and sort it; and we pull together discrete events, statements, and observations. Coding is often the analytical step with which novices are most familiar, even if they don't quite know what it entails.

Analysis is the process of reducing, working with, and distilling data to help answer the question of what to do with the results of our coding. It allows us to order our data, converting large, unorganized data into smaller, summarized sections. Analysis also enables us to discover and connect patterns and themes in the data.

Interpreting data means examining its relationships and patterns to produce an idea of what the research results mean. We reconnect our data to the research question, explaining it through the researchers' and participants' experiences, empirical evidence, and any theories from relevant disciplines. Interpretation often incorporates both *emic* and *etic* perspectives. The emic perspective makes the researcher's story meaningful to insiders and privileges participant meanings; the etic perspective serves to connect the data and the participants' words to larger theoretical disciplinary frameworks generally constructed by the researcher and meaningful to academics or professionals: that is, the discipline at-large.

We present these three elements of qualitative analysis in a linear manner and as something that happens *after* data collection. We present this simplified version even though (per best practice), analysis should parallel data collection in qualitative work rather than commence after data are collected to begin. However, we have found that for instructional purposes, a simplified, stepwise process can keep students from feeling overwhelmed by simultaneous data collection and analysis and provide a structure for how they can engage with the volume of text they have to analyze. This approach can also teach students several specific data management skills as part of the analytic process. In contrast to the clear rules for determining the analytic steps of quantitative methods, the more malleable guidelines for qualitative analysis can leave new practitioners uncertain about how to make meaning from the volume of data generated. In short, students are going to want to know whether they're doing it right—and it can be challenging, particularly within the confines of the classroom, to help them navigate their doubt.

Investigation in qualitative research often begins with uncertainty: the direction the study might take, the most relevant kinds of data, the specific population to contact, the most salient kinds of questions. Studies may begin with one set of research questions or conceptual model or even a hunch about an event or phenomenon that will facilitate understanding of a complex social process—only for the whole concept to fall apart or change once research begins. We understand shifts like these all too well—but the fact that teaching requires *some* structure is another reason why we present these methods in a more streamlined fashion than that by which they are likely to be employed in real-world analysis.

Key concepts

While the following definitions are not universally agreed-upon, we think that conceptual clarity (and some simplicity) can be very valuable for both educators and students.

Code: The label given to a particular piece of data that assigns symbolic meaning to the data. Codes are typically researcher-generated and project-specific (i.e., inductive), although sometimes codes instead reflect existing theories or are imported from a similar project (i.e., deductive). Codes also attribute interpreted meaning to the data for later pattern detection, categorization, and theory-building.

Coding: The process of applying codes to data. Coding is an interpretive act: a researcher summarizes, distills, and condenses data. Thus, the process depends on the constructs, concepts, language, models, and theories that undergird the study.

Theme: A theme represents a level of patterned response or meaning from across the data related to the research questions. Themes are an *outcome* of coding, categorization, and reflection. They can sometimes be the codes themselves, but themes are more often several codes lumped together or new concepts that reflect broader patterns within and insights into the data.

Variable: A category whose component parts vary in a given dimension of the study and is often a tool for comparative purposes within a study. You can also think of a variable as a structural code associated with an entire document.

One of the most common kinds of variables is a demographic category that serves to delineate a population's general characteristics (e.g., age, sex, race/ethnicity, educational level, occupation, income, place of residence, religious identity, political affiliation). For example, a researcher might want to understand how men and women experience and consider illness through the following question: "Do men and women talk about illness in different ways?"

Other types of structural codes and variables include yes/no categorical codes collected for comparison between and among cases. These might include whether a person engages in a specific health behavior like smoking or regular exercise, or whether they live with a particular health problem like diabetes or HIV. The important distinction for qualitative data analysis is that the researcher uses these answers to make comparisons *across* cases relative to other, coded qualitative characteristics.

We've found that qualitative analysis is best taught and learned when students can engage with data, reflect on their experiences, and read published qualitative papers that illustrate the analytic process. These sorts of engagement can also be an important aspect of learning qualitative analysis because the form, content, and style of qualitative papers can vary much more than those of quantitative papers. While there is no substitute for field experience, it isn't always possible to get substantive experience within a course structure, as we've acknowledged previously. When this is the case, you can combine didactic instruction with strategic exercises that simulate meaning-making and reflection, and call upon critical analyses of the literature. Doing so turns the classroom into a setting where your students will learn and practice qualitative analysis skills and obtain a solid understanding of how to conduct qualitative research.

The goals of qualitative data analysis

The goals of qualitative data analysis are as myriad as those of public health itself. Public health students often assume that the goal of a qualitative study is getting people to tell stories and hearing the participants' stated experiences or opinions. This is certainly one approach to conducting qualitative research. But as Box 6.1 highlights, there are many analytic traditions in qualitative research with different goals and different ways of engaging with theory and data. For example, there are traditions that connect participant narratives to broader theoretical, discipline-specific currents. It's therefore important to expose students to a variety of qualitative research products: projects that center on participant perspectives, for example, as well as research intended to produce a grounded theory of a population or phenomenon, and projects that draw on and illuminate discipline-specific theories or debates.

Box 6.1 Qualitative building blocks: Articulating several potential goals of qualitative analysis

---

You may want to review this list with students who are preparing to engage in analysis. Do any of the following goals resonate with them and help them better articulate their analytic plan? (Note that these goals are not mutually exclusive.)

Comprehension. A primary goal of qualitative data analysis is understanding the participants' perspectives, experiences, and beliefs. Doing so involves exploring the meaning and context of the data.

Interpretation. Qualitative analysis intends its interpretation of data to help develop theories or explanations for the phenomena being studied.

Such interpretation involves identifying and making sense of patterns, themes, and relationships within the data.

Contextualization. For explanatory purposes, qualitative data analysis places data in its relevant social, cultural, and historical contexts. This placement helps the researcher understand how the data are shaped by the larger social and cultural systems in which it is embedded.

Validation. Validating the data means checking its consistency, verifying the accuracy of the interpretations, and assessing the findings' credibility to ensure their reliability and trustworthiness.

Communication. The findings of qualitative data analysis must be communicated clearly and in a compelling way. This means presenting data and interpretations—as well as the richness and complexity of that data—in a manner accessible to the intended audience.

Exposing students to a variety of qualitative products and writing styles can illustrate these diverse goals and audiences for qualitative reports. Such products may include the following:

- **Peer-reviewed articles**. Select articles from a range of public-health-oriented journals, including discipline-specific journals, that represent archetypes for presenting both theory and participant voices.
  - Select articles that represent a range of styles, from those that parallel the structure of quantitative articles to those with a more narrative style.
  - Ask students to compare the articles in terms of how they do and don't use theory, use quotes and other data, and how much context they give about the participants, their history, and their society.
- **Reports for a funder or commissioner of the work**. These reports often differ from peer-reviewed articles in that they are longer and feature more description about the setting and program and (potentially) less about published literature or

other research. USAID or CDC program reports are examples common in the public health space. It is helpful to select different program reports—from one-page summaries to thorough documents.

- **Reports for program managers/decision makers**. Reports or policy memos for the people who make decisions about public health programs and policies often focus on takeaway messages, with a bit of additional detail on the findings most useful for decision making. These reports often have less detail on methods.

A course that includes qualitative data analysis should facilitate consideration of the importance of understanding analytic goals, as these goals should shape the analysis. For example, if your analytic goal is bringing together participant stories and experiences to communicate with policymakers, then your analysis may not engage with theory. If, on the other hand, your primary goal is to shape theoretical understanding within an academic discipline, you will need deep theoretical engagement. Importantly, as Box 6.2 emphasizes, theoretically-driven qualitative data analysis is as empirically grounded as qualitative analysis that aims to more descriptively report participants' experiences.

Box 6.2 Myth buster: Qualitative analysis is not just subjective opinion

Students may begin a qualitative course with the belief that qualitative analysis means little more than spouting an opinion. It's our goal that by the end of any of our courses, students will instead be able to understand and appreciate the many differences between armchair theorizing and genuine qualitative analysis that is empirically grounded. These two things are not the same. No matter the specific goal, qualitative analysis requires explicit and focused engagement with the data.

Getting to know your data: Compiling, managing, exploring

One of our essential messages for students is that, per the principles of iterative study design, they should engage with data from an analytic perspective early in the research process—not just after they've collected all of it. The process of extracting meaning from and creating interpretations of the data and going beyond the generation of discussion topics is not always linear. Along-the-way analysis can be formal or quite informal; what matters is that a researcher engages with data while they still have time to modify their design choices and ensure they're asking the right questions and generating appropriate insights along the way.

While the products of qualitative analysis can vary, we emphasize that there are common processes regardless of the final output, the theoretical lens of the research, or the analyst's epistemological stance. Our list of such processes includes the following:

- getting to know the data
- working and playing with the data
- making sense of the data: interpreting it or relating it to theory
- writing about data

It is helpful to provide students with the opportunity to understand qualitative data structure through data management activities early in your course. It's one way of helping them gain familiarity with the data as an object for them to work with and on. For the most effective hands-on analysis class, students will need data to work with. What these data are, though, should vary based on the students' level of expertise and the duration of the course itself.

Giving students opportunities to work with real-world research data can deepen and strengthen their ability to analyze their own study data because it gives them insight into the complexities of data as a whole (rather than, for example, just single interviews). However, it can be challenging to identify a data set for students to use in the classroom that has the necessary ethical approvals and consents to be used for educational purposes. Box 6.3 provides some ideas for potential sources of data to use in a course. Students can work with a subset of the data or an entire data set. For example, in one of our eight-week term courses on data analysis, we assign a subset of full transcripts (approximately four transcripts, 20–30 pages each) that students work with during the first half of the course. In the second half, they work with a full data set (20–25 transcripts) from a real-world research project that has been coded so they can learn and practice analytic strategies that would usually take place after the analyst had become deeply familiar with the data and completed coding. (Typically, students in this course have already been exposed to qualitative concepts and methods.)

By contrast, for an intensive short course on data analysis (16 hours over two days) in which the usual student is a public health practitioner with minimal prior qualitative research experience, we assign six short illness narrative interview transcripts (approximately five pages each) collected for teaching purposes. The transcripts are the result of qualitative interviews in which graduate students were asked to recall the last time they had the flu or a cold, describe their symptoms and the effect that this had on their lives, and what their recovery was like. The small number of transcripts and constrained narrative allow students to learn the basic techniques associated with getting to know data without becoming overwhelmed by the amount of text, complicated ideas, and personal histories typical of interviews from real-world research projects.

We've also taken part in training in which the data set included very short online classified ads. Truncated data such as these are good in that they are available "real-world" textual data and are adequate for familiarizing students with the most basic technical aspects of qualitative data analysis. However, they won't help students develop the close-reading skills and ability to grapple with a participant's story—both of which a proficient qualitative data analyst will likely need.

Box 6.3 Tips and tricks: Example analytic data sets

The following are some of the data sets and sources that we have used for shorter courses and novice researchers:

- Health Experiences Research Network/Health Talk clips and transcripts
- sample data in software packages
- classified ads
- newspaper opinion pieces or blog posts
- interview transcripts from talk shows
- brief interviews collected for teaching purposes (e.g., asking 5–10 students about their most recent illness)

Data sets and sources for advanced courses might include the following:

- students' own data from their research projects (in-progress or completed)
- data from the instructor's project, in which participants consented to use of their data for educational purposes
- public data sets, such as oral histories from the Library of Congress

In addition, you might have your students develop new research questions for existing data or develop and apply codebooks inductively.

After students have data ready to analyze, a good first step is familiarization with that data. We ask students these questions:

- What are the different types of data?
- Why and how were these data collected?
- How many interviews or documents are in the data set?
- Where and from which participants did the data come?

Beyond reading and rereading transcripts, students can familiarize themselves with data by doing the following:

- reading studies' specific aims, project summaries, interview guides, and consent forms
- reviewing data tables on participant characteristics (e.g., demographics, role)
- reading peer-reviewed publications or reports generated using the data
- creating an organizational system for the data, including a filenaming convention (could include sites, participant demographics, type of method employed, date, data collectors)

Teaching how to read data

If knowing one's data is the foundation of data analysis (Hammersley & Atkinson, 2019), then developing that knowledge requires close and repeated readings. It is during the process of familiarization that we get a sense of what is going on in the data, identify patterns and variations, and link these to our existing knowledge of and theories about social phenomena (Hammersely & Atkinson, 2019; Timmermans & Tavory, 2022). The process of familiarization involves both close reading (immersion) and distance (critical engagement) (Braun & Clarke, 2021). Immersion evokes one of the method's core qualities: an appreciation for the emic perspective, one that prioritizes the meaning insiders ascribe to events, relationships, behaviors, and experiences. Critical engagement involves acting deeper questions about the data such as what kind of assumptions participants make when describing the world and how social norms are depicted in the stories participants tell (Braun & Clarke, 2021).

Strategies for teaching qualitative data reading include a focus on close reading, analytic summarizing, and identifying narratives and stories (Ryan & Bernard, 2003). An initial close reading is a chance for students to do the basic analytical work of noticing interesting things and making connections. Knowing how to read data and what to look for can be overwhelming and confusing—particularly for students who are new to qualitative data analysis. They may struggle to establish their sense of what's important and what's worth analyzing. When teaching students to read data coming in from the field, our task as instructors shifts from data *collection*—an experience that generates a certain proximity to the data—to data *analysis*, which simultaneously creates distance from the data and new familiarity with it by putting it into dialogue with other factors, such as existing theories.

Close reading is a word-level strategy in which students learn to look for specific words, phrases, and expressions to get a sense of what people are talking about. Close reading can also focus on chronologies and sequences of events, people mentioned, and specific places. Whereas qualitative outputs often mention themes being identified in or emerging from the data, the relevant issue is where these themes come from. Codes and themes come from the data themselves and are identified by the researcher based on their knowledge of theory, study question, other empirical literature, and the data themselves (Braun & Clarke, 2021). Close reading helps students bracket their preconceptions about what to look for and encourages them to pay attention to what the data are saying.

To practice, give your students a short data excerpt (a few pages of field notes, an excerpt from an interview) and an accompanying list of what to look for as they are reading. The list might include word repetition (words or synonyms that people use often); specialized or Indigenous vocabulary similar to Becker's (1993) classic example of the word "crock"; metaphors and analogies; and linguistic connectors that indicate relationships among things (e.g., "because," "since," "as a result," "if," "then"). For a second close-reading exercise, give students two data excerpts that address the same phenomenon or experience and ask them to compare the texts. Guide them with questions such as, "How is this text different from the preceding text?" and "What kinds of things are mentioned in both?"

Summarizing is the process of reading each transcript to high-light the main experiences and topics that the interview or focus

group covered. Summarizing can help students get to know participants and their stories as a whole rather than through the decontextualized fragments of text that coding generally produces. Understanding participants' whole narratives can, in turn, facilitate deeper insights at later stages of analysis. This task can be done with a structured template (also known as "free form"), in which students are provided with a list of key topics or domains to summarize for each participant. The structured approach can facilitate data comparisons in later analysis. Another strategy is to read full transcripts (or other data types), then summarize each one as a narrative or story without using a template.

Alternatively, you can show your students other ways of summarizing entire interviews and help them decide for themselves how to organize and what to highlight about each datum. At this stage, it's also good practice to encourage students to take notes as they read on anything they find interesting, noteworthy, or surprising. They can include their initial insights and interests in the summary.

Identifying narratives, stories, and accounts. At the other end of the spectrum, the **narrative** approach to reading the data emphasizes seeing participants' experiences from the perspective of a product, cocreated in the interview setting, that reflects the participant's worldview, how they wanted to portray themselves to the interviewer, and how the interviewer elicited a specific narrative and set of experiences from the participant. Whereas novice students will likely find summarizing and close reading easier methods to grasp, narratives and stories may be more appropriate for students with prior experience analyzing data.

Researchers well versed in the principles of a social constructivist approach can focus on the interview as a narrative with their initial read-through. This approach relies upon the idea that the respondent draws from access and reflects on and constructs knowledge in the interview process in response to the situation of the interview. It acknowledges that the interview is a collaboration, one where meanings and their construction depend on the interviewer and interviewee functioning as active agents. Individual narratives on the part of an interviewee are situated within particular interactions (in this case, an interview) and specific social, cultural, and institutional discourses that exist within the interview and beyond. Narratives can function as moral tales, success stories, and ways of explaining individual and cultural identity. Stories provide a mechanism for exploring how social actors frame and make sense of particular sets of experiences. A person's response to an interview question like "Why?" is understood as drawing from a standard set of socially determined responses—for instance, an interviewee asked why he is depressed might respond with "family problems" or give a related answer. Interview participants may present an identity or persona in response to how they want to be perceived or to fulfill their expectation of what the interviewer wants to hear. As social beings, we (including interviewees) are constantly engaging in a process of meaning-making, creating a cohesive narrative that draws on recognizable cultural scripts or explains events by organizing them into a clear beginning, middle, and end consistent with expectations of what makes for a "good story" (Jarvinen, 2000). Students, however, may not instinctively read interviews from this perspective and may need some guiding questions on how to approach an interview from this more critical perspective. Box 6.4 provides a structured set of questions that students can use to help them think about the stories they read in transcripts and how these stories might reveal something about the social world in which participants live.

Box 6.4 Tips and tricks: Introducing students to interview narratives

---

For an initial reading of data in the classroom, students can read transcripts or transcript excerpts, such as responses to individual questions, and try to identify the story as it's constructed by the interviewee (e.g., the beginning, middle, and end, turning points, causative factors) and the cultural scripts the participants draw from to make sense of their experiences. This exercise therefore requires the instructor to identify transcript segments or other data with obvious cultural scripts and clear storytelling.

continued

Box 6.4 *continued*

People with histories of substance use, to give just one example, may call upon the discourse of recovery and therapy to explain their own lives. To give another, participants may explain social success by drawing upon the tropes of by-the-bootstraps hard work and individualism common in American media.

A set of guiding questions can help your students read from this perspective. Possible questions include:

In the transcripts you've read, how do the interviewees present themselves to the interviewer? How do the interviewer's questions shape the story that the interviewees tell?

Choose one of your transcripts and identify a story other than the diagnosis.

- What is this story about?
- What message is the interviewee trying to communicate to the interviewer? Why this story?
- How do the participants characterize themselves? How do they communicate this characterization of themselves to the interviewer— what words, stories, and examples do they use?

The way that social actors retell their life experiences can provide insight into the characters and events central to those experiences. We can analyze narratives in terms of what they reveal about an individual's experience playing a particular social role, as well as the characteristics, turning points, and influences that led them to that role.

- Who are the key actors?
- What are the instances of transformation and turning points?
- What cultural narratives does the interviewee draw on to tell her story?

Teaching qualitative coding

Because coding can be used to engage with qualitative data systematically, it is a concrete process for organizing qualitative data.

Coding has become sufficiently well known within public health such that it is now an expected part of the qualitative analysis process and can signal to consumers (readers/audience for the work) that data were analyzed systematically and rigorously. It is therefore essential that, when teaching coding, you pay attention to the full coding process, from identifying, naming, and refining individual codes in research questions to deciding when coding is complete. At a minimum, you need to dissuade your students from the belief that coding is no more than using software to highlight different sections of interview transcripts or documents. Moreover, students may have heard of qualitative data analysis software but have little understanding of how it works, how it can be used to facilitate analysis, and what the differences are between different software programs. It can be helpful to incorporate a lesson on qualitative data analysis software into your course to set expectations about its role in analysis, as Box 6.5 suggests.

You can integrate qualitative data analysis software into every analytical teaching strategy we outline related to analysis in this chapter, and we encourage you to do so. Increasingly, software—like coding itself—is recognized as an important tool for data management, organization, and deepening analysis. Beyond these helpful uses, it can also create audit trails, help researchers collaborate on analysis, and keep track of each piece of data's individual state of analysis (e.g., whether a particular transcript has been coded and who worked on it).

Box 6.5   Myth buster: Software doesn't analyze your data for you

In just about every course we teach, we encounter students who assume that putting codes into a qualitative software program like NVivo, MaxQDA, or Atlas.ti is all a researcher has to do to get the answer to a given question. Unfortunately, there is no such magic process! At no point during analysis does the software take over; no software is programmed to

continued

> **Box 6.5** *continued*
>
> run an analysis—at least not at the time of writing this text! Qualitative research methods demand that the researcher begin the analysis, perform all functions, and decide how to organize and make sense of the data. Software is best understood as a great tool for organizing and engaging with data, thereby helping the researcher learn, interpret—and answer research questions for themselves.

We teach coding through a multistep process for which each course's level and purpose determine the level of detail and hands-on skill-building we apply at each step. For a high-level overview course designed to familiarize learners with the method's fundamentals and prepare them to critically read qualitative literature, we would include instruction that conveys the purpose and outlines the process of coding, but we would not dedicate time to coding exercises or assignments. By contrast, we would design a qualitative methods course for doctoral students who are intending to analyze their own data so that the course serves to both explain coding as a tool and prepare our learners to do that work through exercises and assignments that allow them to put their knowledge into action.

Step 1: Articulating an analytic plan

Ideally, your coding and your teachings on coding will be grounded in a specific analytical plan. In our experience, asking students to code data without giving them a sense of why or explaining what the research question is creates a scenario in which they feel adrift in the data and as though they do not have an understanding of what to look for when they code. Their difficulty reading transcripts without a clear research question in mind mirrors the tension between the inductive and deductive approaches to qualitative research (see Chapter 4) and the grounded theory approach to qualitative research. And while it is possible to have students who come with a "blank slate" (those who read data without any preconceived questions or specific analytic goals), you and your students may find it more productive to work with a specific, predetermined research question or analytic plan when learning to code qualitative data.

To that end, there are several ways for you to incorporate the development of such a plan into your classroom. At the most basic level, and depending on the data you use, you can present your students with the original research questions, specific aims, or proposal to understand why the study asked its research question. Alternatively, you might present more advanced students with an overview of the data (i.e., contents of a data set, what questions were asked in the interview) and have them identify research questions they think would be interesting and answerable with the data set. From there, your students can select a question or two that they want to focus on and use these questions for the coding and analytic exercises that follow. One note of caution: if students lack a firm understanding of what constitutes a strong qualitative research question, they may need help developing questions consistent with the goals of qualitative research.

After they identify research questions, students can begin thinking about how to answer them with the data. They'll need to consider the data source, along with whose perspectives and experiences it presents. For example, a data set that consists of interviews with patients discussing their experiences and perspectives on a new drug treatment regimen won't enable students to answer questions about provider perspectives, even if the interviews contain information about patient-provider interactions. But you can ask students to identify what they can look for in the data to answer the question: the interview questions they would focus on, or whether a subset of data is especially relevant to their research questions (e.g., women's experiences rather than men's).

Step 2: Generating codes

Because coding is a somewhat simple matter of creating categories and labeling data, teaching coding can, at first glance, seem relatively straightforward. However, as Braun and Clarke (2006), Timmermans and Tavory (2022), and Saldaña (2015) all advise, effective coding is rarely simple. Coding that contributes most productively to the development of insights into the data should go beyond basic description and categorization, aiming instead to capture latent meaning, reach ideas and expressions theoretically and empirically, and make meaning as well as link data to ideas.

It's for these reasons that we typically pair teaching about creating codes with the reading data exercises above. In order to generate codes, students first need to know how to read data—and that means recognizing what is interesting and relevant in it. Novice qualitative researchers and people who take qualitative methods classes to become informed consumers of qualitative work may never get beyond basic descriptive and organizational codes. But students who intend to produce qualitative work should be encouraged to develop skills and strategies that allow for deeper insights through coding and other interpretive methods.

Before teaching students *how* to code, it's important to teach them *why* we code. At its most basic level, coding facilitates the retrieval of data segments categorized under the same code and unites data fragments that can be used to create categories. By linking different data segments under the same code, decontextualizing those data (e.g., removing a paragraph from the original interview transcript), and recontextualizing them with other data (e.g., juxtaposing them with other participants' responses to the same topic or experience), coding allows us to think of data in new ways. From this perspective, coding is a mindful, active process that aims to create connections within the data and between data and ideas from the literature. Coffey and Atkinson (1996) have emphasized the importance of using codes to establish relationships among data and between data and existing knowledge, rather than thinking of coding as a straightforward process.

The exercise in Box 6.6 offers an example on teaching how to generate codes. You might give your students short passages of text—with each passage limited to just a few sentences or a paragraph. Ask students to identify the label they would use for each extract. The passages you choose should contain multiple levels and layers of meaning; it's important that data offer multiple interpretations, as this characteristic reinforces the idea that coding itself is interpretive and analytical, and not an exercise in objectivity. As Saldaña (2015) said, "All coding is a judgment call."

Box 6.6 Tips and tricks: In-class coding exercise

1. Pair up your students. Give each pair a text to read and code.
2. Each student codes the same text.
3. After the students have each generated three or four codes for their texts, have them write a brief code definition for each.
4. Student pairs should compare codes, coding strategies, and code definitions, keeping in mind the size of their passages, the number of codes they generated, the passages they coded, and their code definitions.
5. Have the paired students agree on the definition and use of at least one code.
6. Bring the group back together and, as a class, discuss the process of identifying codes, coding, coming to a consensus with their partners, and the challenges of each process and how to overcome those challenges.

Once the students are comfortable identifying what is being talked about or conveyed in the data, they can begin creating and applying codes to bigger passages. We suggest that students practice this with take-home activities so they will have sufficient time to read the data closely and identify and apply codes thoughtfully. A take-home coding exercise also works well for both novice and advanced students, although the goals and expectations for the exercise will differ for each group. For the former, the assignment can help students develop basic descriptive codes and hone their fluency with the mechanics of coding (e.g., code passages of text rather than single words; use codes throughout the data set; identify analytically meaningful codes). For the latter, a take-home assignment can help your students develop coding strategies that move beyond mere description and surface-level data interpretation and introduce theoretically grounded codes. (For a sample assignment, see Chapter 9.)

You may find it helpful to show your students examples of what they can achieve from a visual and organizational perspective. After all, you can't assume that they've ever seen a fully coded data set, including a well-developed code system with definitions and a data set in which all data are coded. (It's also entirely possible that they'll have never seen a coded transcript!) You can share fully coded data sets from your own projects or coded example transcripts. (Note that to adhere to data privacy protocols, you'll want to ensure that data are not identifiable. Consider the option of displaying these examples rather than distributing them to the class, and ensure that, however you display or share, you are following your institution's ethical regulations and expectations.)

Step 3: Creating codebooks and applying codes

Though students often become proficient at the process of tagging data through the coding process, it can still be challenging for them to explain what they mean by a particular code. It's at this stage where codebook development—including writing code definitions—comes in. The simplicity of a collection of codes and their definitions can be deceptive because a codebook obscures the decision-making involved in defining and applying codes. These decisions include what to include and exclude; the precise meaning a specific word, phrase, or label; and when to use and not use codes.

The difficulty of articulating code definitions can be further exacerbated when the codes themselves derive from common concepts and ideas within public health (e.g., social support, socioeconomic status, family). As with coding itself, giving your students sample code definitions and codebooks can be a good starting point for their understanding of codebook development goals. You might also show your students different ways of organizing codebooks from different projects.

As is so often the case in qualitative research, there is rarely one right way to organize a codebook. Sometimes you'll want to organize code hierarchies with parent and child codes. Other times, code-books are flat—that is, without hierarchical relationships between the codes. Regardless of the approach taken, students need to be able to explain the logic behind their organization and describe its implications. Codebook development works in the classroom and as a take-home assignment; however, ideally, you'll incorporate both above strategies into your assignments so your students have multiple opportunities to practice writing code definitions. As Box 6.7 shows, in addition to examples, it can be helpful to provide students with some general "rules" about what makes "good" codes and code definitions. (Box 6.8 then covers some common coding pitfalls, and how to address them!)

Box 6.7 Qualitative building blocks: Characteristics of good code definitions

- Codes are operationalized: they are defined such that researchers and others can recognize, easily and consistently, the phenomenon in the data to which the code applies.
- Codes have names. Often, these are single terms or short phrases such as "sex," "alcohol," "sharing," "dropping out of school."
- Code names are close to the concepts they describe. "Religion" describes faith in general; subcodes can be more specific (e.g., "Catholic," "Muslim," "Buddhist," "atheist").
- Codes may exist at different levels of abstraction or observation (e.g., "showing respect for elders" is more abstract than "parents").
- Codes can reflect qualities, such as presence, absence, or a degree of presence (e.g., "high," "moderate," "low").
- Generally, codes are not numbers. (However, a code system can be numbered.)
- Code names are distinct from one another.
- Codes when applied are not mutually exclusive—the same block of text can include distinct, intersecting codes. Codes themselves (in concept and naming) should be distinct.

Box 6.8 Qualitative building blocks: Common coding pitfalls (and how to address them)

Some of the most common coding errors include the following:

- descriptive coding as the default
- code proliferation
- coding very small text segments
- overexplaining the presence of a code (which usually suggests that the coder is reading too much into the data)

To deal with the above errors, you may want to apply the following strategies:

- Code as a "lumper", not as a "splitter":
  - Use large units.
  - Use grammatical units as an organizational structure or bounds for coding (e.g., paragraphs, sentences).
  - Use the smallest possible continuous unit (e.g., entire stories, answers from beginning to end).
- Use selected codes often (to aid with pattern detection).
- Remember that codes can and will overlap.
- As you code, subsume codes into broader categories as appropriate.

The dialogic, collaborative practice of developing and defining codes is an important part of the iterative nature of qualitative analysis. You should encourage your students to refine the way they think about their codes and data as they explore them. A code system is never perfect on the first attempt; it often takes many rounds of discussion and revision before a researcher feels confident that their system is comprehensive enough to organize the data and do justice to its range of experiences, expressions, and perspectives.

The iterative process of code definition and codebook development is also a key part of team-based research and analysis. Many students do or will work in teams; the exercise in Box 6.9 is a good way to show them what a consensus-based approach to analysis looks like (see Figure 6.1).

Box 6.9 Tips and tricks: Writing and refining code definitions

For this exercise, you can use the same data set or excerpt you used in the creating codes exercise in Box 6.6.

- Ask students to read and create codes (tags) for the same passage of data.
- Have each student define their codes and apply them to the text, referencing the principles of good code definitions in Box 6.8.
- Put students into pairs and ask them to compare their codes and definitions with their partner. Working together, students should revise the definitions, paying attention to their clarity of terms. The goal is to ensure that the code and its definition could apply to different manifestations of a phenomenon, concept, or experience throughout the data set and to distinguish the codes from each other.
- Have your students share their rewrites with the class and compare how they defined similar concepts and codes. Let this process be the foundation for a guided conversation about the ability to arrive at consensus regarding straightforward, obvious topics in the data and the challenges of doing so when the topic is an abstract or theoretically grounded concept.

You can also have students code a selection of data as a homework assignment, after which they can compare and refine their work in class as previously described. Figure 6.1 illustrates what this process can look like. The image features a table containing every code that

continued

Box 6.9 *continued*

---

three separate analysts generated from the same transcript. Over a series of meetings and conversations, the analysts decided which codes and concepts to merge (i.e., different code names indicated similar topics and concepts), which codes to group because of conceptual similarities, what to retain from each analyst/coder, and topics and concepts to add to or remove from the code system. We find a visual depiction of the process helpful, as in Figure 6.1: it's literal proof for students that developing and refining codes is not necessarily linear and can be very time-intensive.

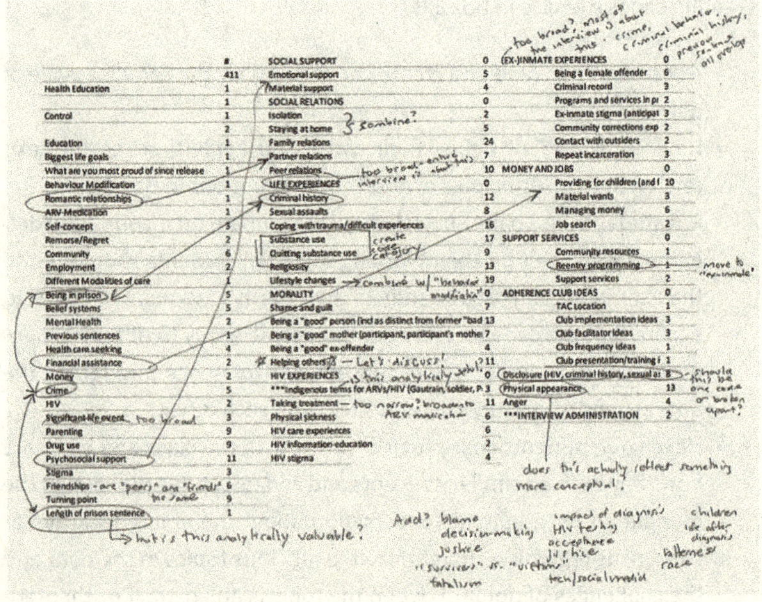

Figure 6.1 Picture of the process of reconciling codes from multiple coders

One struggle is that at some point code development needs to end, and coding needs to begin and eventually be completed! It is possible to iterate and revise a coding plan for eternity, but any faculty member can explain how practical constraints—like time, money, and stakeholder obligations—at some point require us to finalize our code systems and put them to use. There is a point in every project when the researchers and analysts must agree that their system is good enough and that they'll make no further changes. A related question students often have when developing a code system is how many interviews or texts to read when trying to develop a codebook. As with many aspects of qualitative research, the answer to this question is usually, "It depends." We can offer students general guidelines to consider within the context of a particular research project. For example, a more homogenous sample with a set of participants who largely share similar backgrounds and experiences might require the analyst to read fewer transcripts in the process of developing a code system. If a sample is more diverse and includes individuals with vastly different experiences, the analyst would read more transcripts purposefully selected to reflect the range of potential experiences and perspectives that *might* appear in the data and subsequent interviews. In addition, the number of interviews to read to inform the code system might also depend on the level of structure within the interviews—unstructured and open-ended interview questions might produce more diversity of responses than more structured interviews, meaning that more transcripts will need to be read in the former situation.

For more advanced students, these discussions of "how many interviews are enough" could be addressed in a unit on saturation (Guest et al., 2006; Hennik et al., 2019; Lowe et al., 2018; Malterud et al., 2016; Weller et al., 2018). It's important to remind students that no code system will be perfect and any code system will have gaps. Students should be mindful of their own coding decisions and why their code system looks the way it does so they can defend it conceptually and scientifically, feel confident that it will help them achieve their research goals, and know that it reflects the concepts in the data. Finally, more advanced students may also ask about team-based coding and calculating similarity of code application across team members—or inter-rater reliability. Box 6.10 presents our perspective on inter-rater reliability and offers some class exercises on this topic.

Box 6.10 Myth buster: Inter-rater reliability isn't usually central to qualitative analytic rigor

Students and colleagues alike often ask us about inter-rater reliability (IRR), or inter-coder reliability. In general, we do not teach IRR in our qualitative data analysis class as part of an overview course. In fact, we often give it as an example of an attempt at imposing an objectivist paradigm onto constructivist data. However, we recognize that it is sometimes used and may have value, particularly within specific scholarly communities or fields like content analysis, or as a way to signal rigor with more quantitatively oriented audiences.

If you want to include IRR in your course, you have several options, which depend on your teaching goals. To help students consider the pros and cons of using IRR, you might organize a debate on the topic. Divide the class into "for" and "against" camps. To help students prepare, assign them relevant readings on IRR in qualitative data analysis (e.g., Armstrong et al., 1997; Cascio et al., 2019; Morse, 2015; Santiago-Delefosse, 2016). You can also instruct your students to provide peer-reviewed articles that do and don't use IRR and analyze the merits of each author's approach. Then, have the two sides present their arguments and supporting evidence to the full class.

An alternative exercise to help students articulate the epistemological assumptions behind IRR is to have them craft an argument against someone who declares that IRR is a core component of good qualitative analysis. In one analysis class, students were assigned readings that described coding and analysis from a constructivist approach and detailed the link between epistemology and analytic approach. They were then asked to respond to this prompt on the course's Discussion Forum:

> After this class ends, you are very excited to practice and refine your new qualitative data analysis skills. You find a job posting for a research assistant to help with qualitative data analysis. The research is outside your area of specialization, and you weren't involved in the development of the project or data collection. The team is looking to hire a "second coder." You and another student will code all the data with a previously developed coding scheme that consists of mostly semantic and descriptive codes. The research team wants to calculate inter-rater reliability because they believe that is a critical step in producing a rigorous, high-quality qualitative study. The PI asks for your honest thoughts on their proposed approach. Drawing on the perspectives on coding offered by Timmermans and Tavory; Braun and Clarke (Chapter 3; pp. 228–250), what questions would you ask the PI, why would you ask these questions, and what suggestions for alternative approaches might you offer?

This exercise can also help students understand that there are different perspectives on and approaches to qualitative data analysis and identify the links between epistemology, study design, and analysis.

Finally, if you do want to teach students how to actually use and calculate IRR, you can do that! Just remember to include the many nuanced decisions they will need to make—such as how data should be segmented and what statistical test to use.

Teaching meaning-making and data interpretation

Teaching students how to make sense of their data—how to understand the significance of participants' experiences and perspectives and interpret their findings within a broader theoretical, substantive, or disciplinary context—is one of the most challenging aspects of teaching qualitative data analysis. While specific, well-crafted exercises help make it possible to teach them how to read and code data with a basic level of proficiency, we've found that subsequent analytical and interpretive phases often occur without a map.

Moreover, the diversity of academic, theoretical, and experiential backgrounds in a single qualitative data analysis course makes the task of helping all your students understand the significance of qualitative data beyond a single case or descriptive summary even more challenging.

It's important for an analysis course to emphasize that **coding is the beginning—not the end goal—of analysis**. It's therefore advisable to keep this idea in mind when planning your course so that you can allow ample time for students to develop analytical skills beyond coding. Below, we present a few of the ways that you might teach analysis, interpretation, and meaning-making, though we also readily concede that this aspect of qualitative research may be the most difficult to master and to teach. After your students have learned to code data, don't leave them feeling like they must figure out the next part out on their own! Building into your class the time to help them learn what to do with their data after coding will make an enormous difference.

You can consider the use of coded data from two equally valid perspectives: for telling stories and for engaging with and generating theories. An introductory course may focus on using data to generate close, participant-oriented descriptions of an issue; such analysis can be important for work that influences white papers and reports, and advocates and policymakers, and that is shared with community participants. More theoretically oriented and engaged analysis (i.e., that which might be more appropriate for a scholarly or academic audience) would be more appropriate for an advanced qualitative course. In either case, students will need the tools and strategies to make sense of coded data.

Exploring coded data

One way to think about coding is to liken it to the process of separating the raw data into drawers based on common characteristics. To extend the metaphor, then, sense-making is like opening one messy drawer, dumping out all the coded data and reorganizing it such that it now tells the story of the relationship among the newly ordered items (and maybe even makes a connection with the data in the other drawers). Comparing data matrices and tables is one way of sense-making; code mapping and landscaping are others (Miles et al., 2019).

Students may be familiar with the language of themes—the patterns and meanings found across the data. Themes are one product of coding, categorization, and reflection. The strategies below will help students identify and describe themes and help them do more with their data analysis than create lists of topics (a typical pitfall of beginner qualitative analysts).

Exploring using a One-Sheet-of-Paper approach

Effective qualitative analysis involves identifying patterns in the data and realizing how to understand individual experiences in the context of the data set as a whole and in conversation with other participants' experiences and points of view, as well as how core experiences vary among participants. Because this approach to understanding data functions across perspectives, Maietta et al. (2021) have called it a horizontal analysis.

To help instructors teach horizontal analysis, researchers at Oxford University's Health Experiences Research Group (Ziebland & McPhearson, 2006) pioneered OSOP, or the **One-Sheet-of-Paper** approach. OSOP allows the analyst to read through all text segments associated with a specific code and account for the diversity of perspectives of *all* study participants, rather than the most common or most interesting. The goal with this approach is an explanation of "what is going on in the data" (Ziebland & McPherson, 2006). High-quality, rigorous qualitative data analysis requires just such a systematic data evaluation.

In brief, the steps of the OSOP method are as follows:

- Identify part of the data you want to explore (e.g., a single code, the intersections of two or more codes, or the responses to a specific interview question).
- Export/gather all the relevant data.

- Read through each section of data.
- On a single sheet of paper (this is the OSOP approach, after all), note every issue raised in the coded extracts and their corresponding unique ID numbers.
- Group similar responses and issues.
- If one response is similar to an earlier response, add its ID number to that response.
- Record everything, even if it's repeated.
- Create new groups/categories as new issues arise.

Creating an OSOP will result in a summary of all issues within the code and their accompanying ID numbers. With this information, you can explore how the issues connect, how they form broader themes, or the characteristics that connected participants share. In addition, while OSOP was developed to be completed by hand, it is easily adapted to qualitative data analysis software (see Figure 6.2).

Exploring by creating memos

Much of the process of developing insights and drawing meaning from participant experiences comes from writing throughout the stages of engagement: notes taken during interviews, summaries of field experience, and formal write-ups of study findings. Qualitative researchers are encouraged to make notes, jottings, memos, and comments throughout the research process, from their initial reading of transcripts through coding and reading segments of coded text. Doing so helps raise questions, capture initial insights, document reflections, and elaborate on ideas. Charmaz (1999) has considered memos essential for moving from analysis to writing—it's a mechanism that focuses thought on the data. Memos can be a rapid, informal conceptual epiphany or a question about the data; they include elaborate, extended narratives about emerging patterns, categories, theories, emergent theory, and connections with existent theory or research. Furthermore, this writing can also document analytic decision-making.

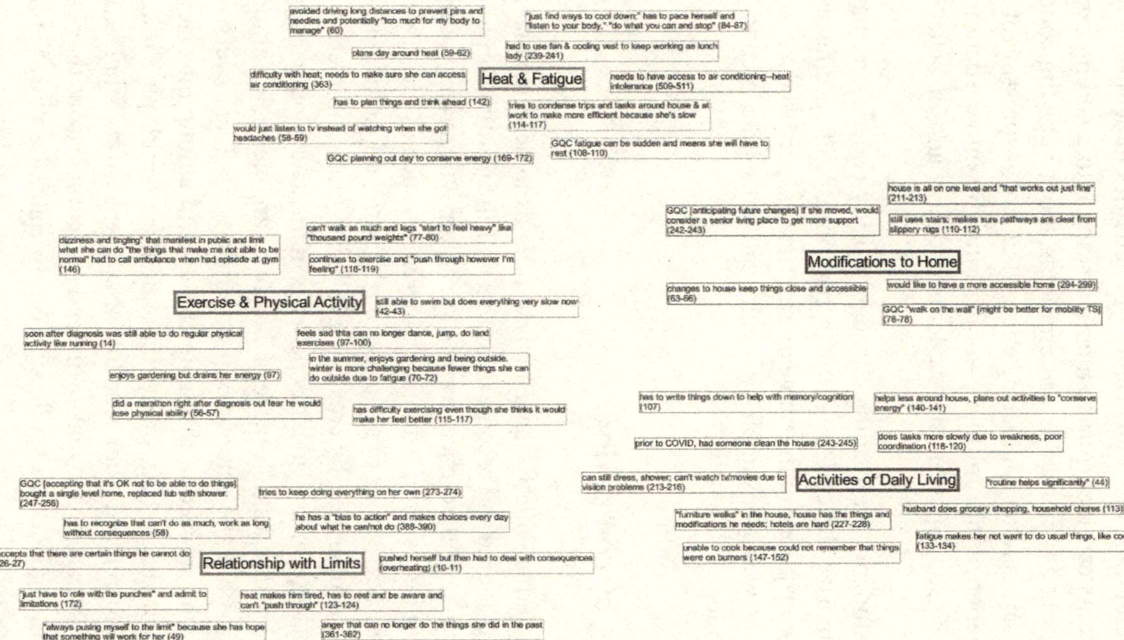

Figure 6.2 An OSOP (One Sheet of Paper) data analysis strategy, completed in MAXQDA, that explores how MS affects people's personal lives

In your course, you can simply explain writing-as-analysis—or you can go further and support students as they develop this skill. In the latter case, there are many classroom activities to help students learn. Students can incorporate memo writing into a coding exercise, recording any questions or comments about applying codes, their observations after comparing one participant's expression of an idea or experience with another's—or their insights into the data and whether they support what the students had read and/or believed beforehand.

If your students are reading through already-coded data, have them summarize the coded text with paraphrases of specific segments or descriptions of the range of experiences, perspectives, and responses, as well as examples of each segment within a code or group of codes.

Exploring by comparing

As we've stated, qualitative data analysis intends to decontextualize data from its source and recontextualize it within an entire corpus of data, literature, or theoretical frames. As an analytic strategy, comparisons can be a way of exploring differences, such as identifying different perspectives or experiences of the same phenomenon; of considering similarities, by creating a fuller or more complete picture; and of beginning to identify patterns in the data. Comparisons are possible within a single piece of data (e.g., an interview), among interviews within the same group of participants (e.g., everyone in a study who worked at the same clinic), and among interviews from different groups (e.g., every respondent from multiple clinics). Remember to remind your students that there isn't a single correct set of comparisons to make—indeed, the comparisons they can make within a given data set depend on the data, the study's aims, and the questions.

There are several ways for you to incorporate comparative reading exercises into your classroom. Students can identify two pieces of data from different participants (either entire transcripts or excerpts), then read each piece of data looking for similarities and differences in how the participants experienced or interpreted a phenomenon. Students can also read coded text segments divided by participant type for consistencies and inconsistencies within the group and similarities and differences with other groups. In any exercise, you should support your students in paying attention to what appear to be typical experiences, what appears to be unusual or unique to a particular group, and to any themes, concepts, or experiences that cut across groups or cases.

Exploring using matrices

Data matrices, or data displays with rows and columns, can be a useful organizational tool, helping bring coherence to what can seem like an overwhelming, cumbersome jumble of unstructured data: field notes, interview transcripts, and all manner of other documents. Miles et al. (2019) have noted that "displaying your condensed data in a systematic way … requires you to think about your research questions and what portions of your data are needed to answer them." Data matrices are also a key component of the framework method for management and analysis of qualitative data using a thematic approach (Gale et al., 2013). A matrix's rows and columns will vary based on the research project and questions. Box 6.11 provides an example of how you might introduce matrices in your classroom.

Box 6.11 Tips and tricks: Creating data matrices

If students have coded data to work with, you can have them create matrices from it. One possibility is a participant-by-code matrix, as shown in Figure 6.3. A participant-by-code matrix displays summaries of

continued

Box 6.11 *continued*

coded data for each person interviewed and provides the researcher with a ready comparison of data across participants. For this exercise, you would ask your students to summarize either a few codes or just one (depending on time) and to then create a table in which each row represents a participant, and each column is a code. They can then fill each cell with their summary of the participant's experiences associated with that code.

Documents	Parenting with MS	Lessons and Insights	Thinking about the future
Participant 1	still able to be a scout troop leader and do things with sons; kids didn't "feel sorry for me," which would have been "the worst thing of all."	accepts things he can't change, "do the best I can."	Sense that no one can answer questions about the future and how disease will progress: "I've never really gotten any answers on before I started physical therapy is whether if you lose, like, strength, or if you lose neurological capability, whether or not that's something that can be restored." Sense of uncertainty about the future: "Will I have to at some point start using a wheelchair?" WIll he need to make modifcations to the house.
Participant 2	worried about the effects of pregnancy on MS but doctor	"not like Pollyanna" and sees that other people are worse off.	describes thinking about the future as "terrifying." Doesn't

Documents	Parenting with MS	Lessons and Insights	Thinking about the future
	assured her it would be fine. Had two kids. Had a babysitter for kids "seamless childcare." Kids take on role of supporter. Need to use support systems and ask for help (carpools, help from neighbors) especially if have limited mobility	She's "just glad I can still eat, speak, enjoy my kids, enjoy my husband. I love this town we live in. And we've never had money problems."	know what the effects of being sedentary (in a wheelchair) will be. Worries what she would do if something happened to her husband. "It's very fragile." wants to stay in house as long as possible
Participant 3	feels like he is missing out because he can't do things with daughter like hik	Painting has given him meaning and purpose: "I can say that 'inability is the new ability for me.'	Uncertainty about the future, lack of control. Fear about future but has to change attitude and "live it for today I have left the thought of tomorrow."
Participant 4	questioning what it would mean to be a father and getting to a place where focusing on what he can do rather	"Resilience is a skill" and has a lot of help.	after diagnosis, concern about the future in the sense of "What if this ist it? What if this is how I'm going to feel for the rest of my life?"
Participant 5	challenge of managing the process of getting diagnosed (e.g., doctor's visits) with being a single parent.	had to learn to "give up the control" and "let things go." Taught her that she "can't give up." "Life is a long journey of just learning."	after she realized disease was not progressisng, was able to start making goals and overcome the feeling that ms diagnosis "stopped

continued

Box 6.11 *continued*

Documents	Parenting with MS	Lessons and Insights	Thinking about the future
	after getting diagnosis, worried about what that would mean for daughter in terms of who would take care of her if she were disabled, not wanting to hide condition from her.	me" ["for a year, I just had no goals"]	

Figure 6.3   Example of a participant-by-code data matrix

Conceptualizing data

The strategies above are useful when helping students develop their ability to *describe* data and create a systematic description of the relationships between essential aspects *of* the data. But another aspect of qualitative data analysis is *interpreting* these data—understanding their meaning. Interpretation can occur at multiple levels, including making sense of a particular social context or case (e.g., explanatory models, theories of the data) and linking findings to discipline-specific concepts (e.g., social science theories) or overarching worldviews (e.g., feminism, Marxism). Conceptualization is best understood as creative intellectual work requiring the analyst to develop conceptually dense accounts that incorporate all observed cases and that capture key features of the given phenomenon. Classroom instruction and assignments on this topic should give students a chance to manipulate data and the products of analysis (e.g., code systems, data summaries), then talk through or write up what they notice and conclude.

Some learning activities for conceptualization include the following:

- **Reorganize code systems into categories**. Begin by categorizing initial codes both concrete (e.g., people) and conceptual (e.g., political ideologies). Next, name the categories. Then, reorganize them to create a network or diagram that demonstrates how the codes relate to each other.
- **Answer a research question**. Propose a question related to a data set with which the students have been working. Have them create a model of the data to answer the question before returning to the data to identify examples and quotes that illustrate and support the case.

Ideally, this exercise would also identify and include negative cases or contradictory evidence in the model. Conversations about the data and an instructor who encourages dissent and counterexamples will help correct for the tendency to overemphasize patterns in data and exclude evidence that might not fit, allowing students to revise their data models and deepen their understanding of the phenomenon. Another strategy for exploring data that embraces contradictory or surprising findings is the index case strategy (Timmermans & Tavory, 2022), detailed in Box 6.12.

Box 6.12 Tips and tricks: Exploring an index case

Timmermans and Tavory (2022) proposed the strategy of "index cases" for anchoring your empirical and analytic narratives (p. 10). These cases should exemplify one of your insights into the data, or preliminary theories or models about a particular aspect of the data. It's for this reason that an index case is not necessarily the average case; instead, "what renders an index case effective is that it makes a theoretical point that clarifies

continued

> **Box 6.12** *continued*
>
> ---
>
> other excerpts and thus allows us to launch into a promising analytical line of coding" (p. 110). Students can complete an index case exercise in-class, as a take-home assignment, or as an online discussion forum post.
>
> To begin, students should think about their data and select a potential index case. Then, have them describe the case and explain why they chose it. What does this example reveal about the data or a larger phenomenon? After this, students can write a research or analytic question about their index case such that they recontextualize the instance within the broader data set. The next step is identifying a theoretical framework for analyzing the data, beginning with the index case. The final step is a summary of that theory and an explanation of how it would guide their analysis. What questions would they try to answer through their analysis? How would their chosen theory illuminate the data? How might their data complicate the theory?

Interpretative power

In our advanced courses, we dedicate time to discussing the power dynamics of analytic interpretation. Throughout our qualitative courses, we engage repeatedly with the concept of the researcher as a crucial instrument of the research, which therefore means that they can't be considered a neutral factor in the conduct of that research or the nature of the data it generates. The researcher's position likewise influences the analytic process—the person interpreting the data and doing the meaning-making has considerable power over the story that the data will tell. This is not to say that the researcher is nefarious or intends to skew the analytic focus in any direction, but there is power in meaning-making. Thus, we should be mindful about the person with whom that power sits, how they came to be positioned this way, and the possible implications of having their perspective at the fore.

It is a valuable exercise to ask students to ask the following questions about their own research, as well as any other research they encounter:

- To the extent that qualitative analysis is a process of meaning-making—who is doing the meaning-making in the research?
- Is there any way that the participants' perspectives can contribute to (or even lead) the meaning-making process?
- Does someone with lived experience lead the research?
- Is there anyone with lived experience on the research team?
- Is there any mechanism for checking interpretation with those who have lived experience?
- How has the researcher optimized their understanding of the research setting or phenomenon?
- Does the researcher (or members of the research team) engage with and present their positionality in relation to the subject of study?

By this point, it will probably come as no surprise to hear that we also explain there isn't one right choice to undertake in any research project or lead analysis. It's simply always important to consider the effect of the perspectives of those doing the research. There are benefits to an emic perspective, just as there is insight to be gained from the etic viewpoint. Is it possible to construct an analytic approach that integrates both?

Every researcher needs to understand the perspectives they bring to the analytic table and the influence they have. It is through this acknowledgement that the audience for their research can understand these factors too. Self-reflexive insight should be an important factor in their assessment of the interpretation. Bringing this dynamic into the classroom can increase students' ability to interpret and disseminate contributions from qualitative research.

Analytic saturation

Frequently, our students ask, "How do you know that you are done with analysis? How do you know that you have it right?" These questions are not easy to answer. We find it helpful to acknowledge the struggle with our students. Saturation is one criterion that qualitative researchers use when deciding whether to stop data collection and analysis (Saunders et al., 2018). The concept is not, however, easy to define—it relates to many aspects of the research process, and there are just as many ways to conceptualize it. Asking the following questions can help determine analytic saturation:

- Does the researcher *really* know what they need to know?
- Are they gathering new (pertinent) information from new data collection?
- Has an interviewee shared all that they have to share?
- Are there new codes or other useful labels to apply to the data, or do the new data only provide more examples to existing codes?
- Does the researcher understand the relationships and connections between the codes and know how to make sense of the data in this form?

Transfer of knowledge

The goal of qualitative research is rarely to generalize the knowledge from a single study sample for a broader population. Instead (as outlined in Chapter 1), its goal is usually to transfer or apply the findings and insights of one study to situations that share meaningful characteristics. The transfer of insights or theory is often considered the work of an individual reader or of a study's audience. And while this is indeed the case, it's also true that much about the study's presentation will facilitate or hinder the growth of these connections. Analysis that outlines *why* a particular finding occurs or *how* a process works can be written in to inspire and inform future research for the researcher *and* for the reader.

Teaching with computer software packages

The decision of how to teach with qualitative data analysis software (QDAS) or whether to use it at all is one you'll have to make for your own course in alignment with the course's learning objectives, the broader curriculum in which the course is situated, and any institutional or accreditation requirements. For example, the Council on Education for Public Health (CEPH) includes among its Master of Public Health foundational competencies, "Analyze quantitative and qualitative data using biostatistics, informatics, computer-based programming and software, as appropriate." This competency may be interpreted to mean that students are taught to use a specific software program (a dedicated QDAS) or something general (like Word). In the real world, QDAS is widespread; many research teams use it in a variety of settings and for a variety of projects. QDAS has tremendous data management and analytic capability, and its potential, already under constant expansion, is likely to grow even more with advances in generative artificial intelligence. Bringing QDAS into your classroom will allow your students to become familiar with it and its creative problem-solving capabilities for a range of analytic goals.

On the other hand, incorporating QDAS into your teaching means you first need to decide *which* software program to use. "QDAS" is a general term for all qualitative data analysis software; it isn't a software package unto itself, and there is no gold-standard QDAS. You can encourage students to make informed decisions about whether and which software programs to use by incorporating an activity or assignment into your course in which students compare the trial versions of different programs, as described in Box 6.13. When studying the specifics of (to name only a handful of examples) MaxQDA, Atlas, NVivo, Dedoose, or any other possible options, you'll need to consider familiarity, cost, aesthetics, institutional access, and functionality, among other factors. And should you decide to include your students in the selection (a not-unreasonable possibility, given that this could be their first exposure to QDAS and could turn out to be foundational for their careers), you'll want to remember that most software programs are not interoperable. Practically, what this means is that it won't be possible for your students to share files, data, coding, or analytic products with anyone using different software. Finally, incorporating QDAS means you risk bogging down class sessions with the minutiae of technical assistance and troubleshooting.

Regardless of your QDAS decision, you should reiterate to your students that software does not do the thinking for them any more than a power saw can map out how to cut down a tree or cut a tree down itself. It is a tool to help manage and organize data and may help with generating summaries—no more.

Finally, here's a short list of helpful QDAS features:

- inter-rater reliability scores (remembering our skepticism of the utility of these for qualitative analysis)
- code frequencies and associations between codes
- data visualizations
- audit trails
- data management and tracking

Box 6.13 Tips and tricks: Software comparison exercise

Students and researchers may be asked for advice about QDAS by colleagues looking to make a purchase. Whether or not you use QDAS in your classroom, you can help your students become informed consumers by having them compare different options. For this exercise, they'll download trial versions of two different software programs and explore each one: the features, tools, and user interfaces, and any other characteristics you deem important. In a class discussion forum or a written response, ask your students to describe the similarities and differences they see, along with each program's ease of use and interface options, and their own preferences.

(Each QDAS platform has overview and demonstration videos for their software; many of these videos are also available on YouTube. You might find these helpful when working on this exercise.) An additional component to this exercise would be to have students code by hand (or in a nonspecific word processing program like Microsoft Word or Excel) and then by using QDAS, followed by a discussion or written reflection that considers the strengths and benefits of each approach.

Artificial intelligence and qualitative data analysis

As we write this book, artificial intelligence (AI) is taking off all over society. Qualitative research is no exception. Some QDAS packages now incorporate AI tools to generate text summaries (in memo form) and code data. Several of them also allow the analyst to ask questions of the data in a conversational format. While we cannot predict AI's future role in qualitative research, we anticipate that it will be substantial. Even now, AI can sometimes do a decent job summarizing qualitative data. Simple summaries and descriptive analysis may be all that some research projects need, so using AI to these ends may be what some students need to learn to meet their learning goals.

You might encourage students to play around with AI tools for qualitative data analysis and compare them with the analysis they can do themselves. What is AI good at? What doesn't it do so well? What are its weaknesses? When might your students consider using it? What do they consider the ethical issues associated with AI use? How might AI's incorporation into qualitative research reshape who we collaborate with—for example, would we still want an expert in large language models on the research team?

Summary

Students may struggle with the concepts and strategies of qualitative analysis and interpretation, and they may express discomfort with the sometimes-tenuous processes of meaning-making with and through data. Their struggles are understandable when we remember that these concepts and strategies are also some of the hardest things for us to teach. And the classroom allows us not just to tell students what to do, but to *show* them the mechanisms by which the researcher engages with data, organizes it, focuses on key elements, and builds meaning. Because, of course, the best way for students to understand qualitative analysis is to do it themselves.

We appreciate Patton's (2002) wise words: "Qualitative inquiry ... works best for people with a high tolerance for ambiguity." Ambiguity aside, we hope that this chapter has given you some concrete ideas for breaking down the numerous steps of analysis and helped you see how to demystify the process while appreciating its flexibility.

Additional readings on qualitative data analysis

The following is a list of resources that you and/or your students may find to be particularly useful as grounding for aspects of the analytic approaches outlined in Chapter 6.

- Braun, V., & Clarke, V. (2006). Using thematic analysis in psychology. *Qualitative Research in Psychology*, *3*(2), 77–101.
- Cascio, M. A., Lee, E., Vaudrin, N., & Freedman, D. A. (2019). A team-based approach to open coding: considerations for creating inter-coder consensus. *Field Methods*, *31*(2), 116–130.

- Miles, M., Huberman, A., & Saldaña, S. (2019). *Qualitative data analysis: A methods Sourcebook* (4th ed.). Sage Publications.
- Saldaña, J. (2015). *The coding manual for qualitative researchers* (3rd ed.). Sage Publications.
- Timmermans, S., & Tavory, I. (2022). *Data analysis in qualitative research: Theorizing with abductive analysis*. University of Chicago Press.

7

Teaching Ethics, Rigor, and Reflexivity

Many things go into designing, conducting, and analyzing a qualitative study, beyond considerations of where to go, whom to talk to, or even specific methods for collecting data. It is critical to consider how to *do* ethical and rigorous research and to be deliberate in our consideration of how we, as researchers, engage with participants and communities. The process of "performing scientific research in human beings or with human beings implies respecting the dignity and liberty of participants, which is crucial to ensure the integrity and quality of the study," and that process requires intention (Taquette et al., 2022). In this chapter, we outline our thoughts about and approaches to addressing these necessary elements in qualitative methods courses. Of course, the issues we cover in this chapter are not exhaustive; they are simply those with which we engage most routinely in our own courses.

To be competent consumers and producers of qualitative research, students need to understand the following:

- **Qualitative studies' unique ethical issues**. We assert that ethics is a necessary component of any qualitative research course.
- **What makes a high-quality qualitative study**. Considerations of **rigor** are important and often touch upon the foundational differences between qualitative and quantitative approaches.

Teaching Qualitative Research in Public Health. Katherine Clegg Smith et al., Oxford University Press.
© Oxford University Press (2026). DOI: 10.1093/9780197662472.003.0007

- **How a study is shaped by the people conducting it, and the context in which they conduct it**. These contextual considerations make it important to introduce and engage with the concept of **reflexivity** in qualitative research and analysis.

Consider the following sample of learning objectives pertaining to ethics, rigor, and reflexivity taken from one of our syllabi:

- Anticipate the possible ethical complexities of conducting research that is often iterative, usually in-depth and small-scale, and where a crucial element is the rapport between the researcher and research subjects.
- Articulate why concepts traditionally related to rigor—including objectivity, reproducibility, and generalizability—do not necessarily transfer to qualitative research.
- Describe indicators of rigor that are specific to qualitative research.
- Explain the concept of reflexivity and why it is important for qualitative research.
- List several reflexive practices that can improve qualitative research rigor and ethics.

Ethics

Students are sometimes surprised to find that we prioritize ethics so much in our qualitative methods courses. The general opinion seems to be that ethics is its own topic rather than one to be folded into a methods course. However, unethical research cannot be good research. Therefore, any course designed to support students in conducting rigorous, worthwhile qualitative research, as well as those that teach students how to be good consumers of qualitative literature, should pay attention to the ethical concerns that may arise during qualitative research studies. By including ethics in our methods courses, we give students opportunities to consider how they might respond to an important decision or determination in the real-world scenario and to appreciate how ethics affects the methods decisions that qualitative researchers make.

It is more difficult to react appropriately in the moment when you find yourself confronted by a scenario totally new to you. Taquette et al. (2022) observed that because "qualitative research is a dynamic process, and unpredictable events can occur," it is important that the qualitative researcher prepare for ethically important moments by trying to "foresee possible hinderances and prevent them from happening" (p. 1).

One way to think about the various ethical considerations of a research endeavor is by differentiating between procedural ethics and ethics in practice (Guillemin & Gillam, 2004). **Procedural ethics** encompasses the norms, standards, and procedures of planning for and conducting ethical work. Such procedures often center on (and go well beyond) gaining Institutional Review Board (IRB) approval and conducting research based on an approved protocol. By contrast, **ethics in practice** relates to the questions and issues that inevitably arise in the conduct of the work—the "ethically important moments" that we refer to above. To provide students with a good grounding in both areas, you'll likely present some key information, along with the chance to engage with their own perspectives and those of others on critical topics.

Qualitative research often raises ethical questions that differ from survey, experimental, or intervention research. You can highlight these differences and their consequences in the context of study design and methods components of your course. For instance:

- Qualitative research design is often iterative, with less formal and predetermined structure than quantitative approaches. A related ethical question is therefore whether the researcher offers sufficient description of their research and analysis for potential participants to provide truly informed consent. As you discuss iterative design, you might raise procedural and practical ethical questions posed in relation to an effective consent process.

- One strength of qualitative research is its smaller scale. Another is that it accounts for the historical, political, social, and economic contexts in which people live. And a third is that it values the rich details and narratives of individual experiences. However, this degree of specificity can create challenges for preserving the confidentiality and anonymity of study participants at the individual and community levels. Will people or organizations be identifiable in the data? Do participants understand that they might be identifiable? What are the potential implications of a participant or locale being identifiable? As you introduce students to interview transcripts and transcription processes, you might have them consider the vulnerabilities of data that are not blinded. What is the right balance of specificity and identifiability when you consider that the participants' rights are at least as important as the study objectives?

- The informal and extended interactional style of some qualitative researchers and methods (for example, ethnography) can blur the boundaries between researcher and participant and contribute to confusion about the purpose of research interactions. When a researcher is embedded in a social setting, they will develop relationships and may become understood to be part of the community. In turn, members of that community may engage with them differently. While this is indeed the intent of the method, a question emerges: what is the researcher doing to maintain boundaries between their work and their relationships over time? In considering this question, we sometimes discuss works that have become known for challenges on this topic, including:

  - Goffman, A. (2014). *On the run: Fugitive life in an American city.*
  - Venkatesh, S. (2008). *Gang leader for a day: A rogue sociologist takes to the streets.*

These books, though now somewhat dated, are valuable case studies of dissertation research that were touchstones for ethical debates related to the appropriate stance of the novice researcher.

Any methods course, qualitative or otherwise, needs to introduce processes related to the ethical review of a research plan. In Box 7.1, we provide some ideas for how to set up a discussion of critical ethical issues. It is valuable to allow students to consider their own reactions to various ethical scenarios and how these reactions may or may not align with institutional expectations or professional norms. Should you facilitate such considerations, you'll also want to give your students time for independent reflection and/or to structure opportunities for group discussion of their reactions. We find it helpful to have our students ponder how they would respond to a study's potential ethical challenges and to then think about how others may see the issue differently. Rarely is there a single right or wrong answer to an ethical question that comes up in a study—although there may be only one course of action acceptable to a student's committee or a school's IRB. Here, we list a few research areas for which qualitative approaches generally raise somewhat distinct ethical considerations and suggest strategies for incorporating them into a course.

Ethical consideration: Can too much rapport ever be a bad thing?

In qualitative studies, we often challenge the idea that it is possible to erase human interactions when conducting research. Research is an interactional experience: the researcher and the researched will necessarily affect one another. Given this, rapport is frequently cited as a factor in enabling high-value data collection. At its core, building rapport means establishing a positive connection between the researcher and the participant, one that helps research subjects feel comfortable in the interaction; since comfortable people provide better data, rapport in turn benefits the research.

An ethical issue you might wish to present to your students is whether there are times when building rapport might blur the lines of voluntary consent. Is it possible that the researcher is seen as a friend or counselor rather than someone whose primary goal is to learn from or about participants? We ask students to remember that, in some instances, establishing very good rapport might eventually result in unmet expectations on the participant's part, or lead either the researcher or participant to engage with topics that go beyond the study's scope and are more emotionally, politically, or socially challenging than anticipated.

The tension between voluntary consent and rapport building is certainly relevant at the beginning of a research study. Will people who feel a connection with someone feel more compelled to participate? The possibility of rapport's influence on voluntary participation continues throughout the study. Qualitative research sometimes entails extended time in the field. If, as time passes, a researcher-participant relationship starts to look a lot like a friendship, it may be that a participant feels less able to stop participating or question what is being asked of them. They might even feel an expectation to share information or other private access where before the relationship they would not have.

Box 7.1 Tips and tricks: Debating ethical dilemmas

In both introductory and advanced classes, you can present students with you and your colleagues' real-world ethical dilemmas or scenarios you think your students may encounter in the field. After you explain a scenario, have your students engage in a think-pair-share exercise on what they, as researchers, would do in that situation. They can discuss the ethical positions that would lead them to a particular action or conclusion. In each case, invite the students to ask the following two questions:

- What is the ethical dilemma?
- What would you do and why?

continued

Box 7.1 *continued*

In our teaching, we've used examples such as:

- After sharing information in an interview, a participant later decides they should not have shared so much. They tell you, "Just delete that" (Janesick, 2016). What do you do?
- You are interviewing frontline staff and the director of a health care clinic for a study. This study required approval from the director, who gave you the staff's contact information and allowed them to take time from their workday to converse with you. After you spend the morning conducting interviews, the director calls you into her office to ask you how the interviews are going and what you're learning. What do you tell her?
- You learn about some problematic practices at a health care clinic during an interview with a staff member. What do you do? Do you inform anyone? If so, who?

Ethical consideration: How do you provide informed consent for a study with an iterative design?

Informed consent is a cornerstone of contemporary ethical research conceptualizations. In qualitative research, the way we do our work can lead to challenges related to informed consent. Because qualitative research is often intentionally iterative, decisions related to sampling and plans for questions to be posed and data to be gathered develop over time. This flexibility allows for adaptation based on emerging data and is therefore a strength. Iterative design can also pose challenges for external consideration and oversight from an IRB, or from other organizations (such as a Community Advisory Board) or even an individual participant. How can a potential participant understand what they're consenting to if the study process or parameters are insufficiently defined?

We devote an entire class of an advanced course on ethnographic fieldwork and participant observation to issues of informed consent. Ethnographic work tends to be iterative and relatively unstructured; the researcher's primary role is that of a participating observer. This class session takes place typically toward the end of the course, after students have been able to familiarize themselves with the realities of participant observation. Challenges reviewed include personal identity issues, relationships with individuals and communities in the field, informing people what the researchers are doing, obtaining consent, and expectations of privacy in different contexts. The students read the American Anthropological Association's Code of Ethics, IRB guidance for required elements of a consent form, and example consent forms for studies approved by the school's IRB. They then engage in small group discussions that explore the following:

- how recruitment and enrollment are conceptualized in an ethnographic study and how this might differ from other types of qualitative or quantitative studies
- ethical considerations of enrollment in ethnographic fieldwork
- who is considered a participant in ethnographic studies and how ideas about inclusion and exclusion criteria may differ for ethnography
- how issues of community and individual risk and harm apply and manifest in ethnographic research
- who should provide consent (i.e., individuals, community leaders) for participation in ethnographic research
- the nature of informed consent as a process, not a one-time occurrence to fulfill IRB requirements (procedural ethics), and what informed consent looks like in practice (e.g., consent is obtained each time an interaction occurs—"Is it okay for me to shadow you today?")

Ethical consideration: Do you need to get informed consent for research conducted in public spaces?

Compared to much experimental and quantitative research, qualitative research is often conducted by the researcher when they go out into the real world seeking to understand how and why things happen. It's not always clear, when a researcher is mid-study, how they might obtain informed consent. The concept of informed consent, itself at the heart of modern ethical research principles, is based on the importance of voluntary research participation. But is it always possible to get informed consent for *public* observational research (see Figure 7.1)? In this case, is such consent necessary? Do you need to get permission from every person in a given space, or are there times when a gatekeeper's permission is enough? If a researcher spends an extended period in the field, is asking permission one time enough? Can there ever be a case for ethical *covert* research, in which a researcher does not disclose their research objectives and/or themselves? See Box 7.2 for ideas about an in-class exercise around ethical issues that can arise in relation to conducting observational research in public spaces.

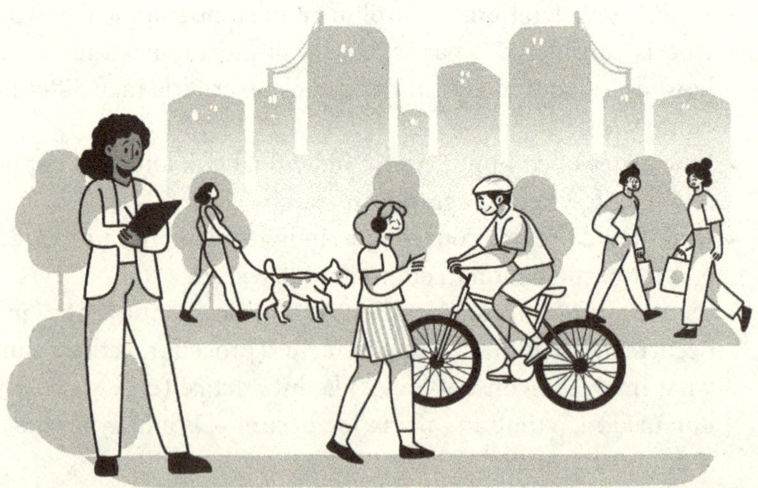

Figure 7.1   It is not always clear if and how informed consent should be obtained in relation to research in public settings

---

Box 7.2 Tips and tricks: Considering consent and privacy in public settings

---

Debate a challenging and relevant ethical issue: is it necessary to get informed consent for research conducted in public spaces? The issue lends itself well to a debate between students and groups who either support or oppose the need for permission for research conducted in public spaces. Before the debate begins, make sure you give students time to consider the issue and prepare a position. It may also be helpful to give them different scenarios—where the research is being conducted, who is conducting it, what they are observing, and the like—and see how your students change their arguments, if they do at all. An instructor-facilitated debrief can be very useful to complete this exercise.

Ethical consideration: How do you keep information-rich data anonymous?

The rich, context-specific nature of much qualitative work can create challenges regarding anonymity. Rigor in qualitative research often means gathering, analyzing, and presenting rich data from well-chosen cases; frequently, context is also key to analytic engagement. But valuing (and therefore retaining), for example, an individual's way of speaking and phrasing may make an anonymized transcript identifiable. And the use of pseudonyms, while important, may not be sufficient to conceal an identity. Furthermore, to facilitate evaluation of the analytic process, we try to provide our readers with access to elements of the raw data in our dissemination. All of these elements can lead to concern that our research participants may lose their anonymity, which we never intend, and which is never appropriate. Careful consideration of when participants might be identifiable, and the implications of this visibility, is necessary for conducting ethical qualitative research. You might ask your students whether there are circumstances under which removing someone's name from a transcript is insufficient to conceal their identity.

Ethical consideration: Power dynamics between researchers, participants, and communities

So far, we've focused our discussion of ethics somewhat narrowly: on the small-scale, interpersonal interactions and dilemmas that can challenge the guiding ethical principles as defined by the Belmont Report (National Commission for the Protection of Human Subjects of Biomedical and Behavioral Research, 1978) and other foundational documents. We can also think about research ethics on a broader scale—which is particularly relevant given the recent attention to the histories of inequitable power dynamics and exploitation in research.

First, it is always important to consider power dynamics between researchers, participants, and communities. We have found that it is not hard to draw attention to historical ways in which inequitable distribution of power has led to harms to individual research participants—as in the famous Tuskegee untreated syphilis experiment—or to whole communities—as evidenced by decades of deficit-framed (instead of strengths-based) research with Native American communities. A simple, "Who benefits and how?" question is often enough to start this discussion.

Recent scholarship documents that our unchallenged assumptions about participants, research questions, methodological choices, and the products of research are rooted in the dominant power structures responsible for marginalizing and exploiting minoritized and colonized groups. Efforts to decolonize research methods aim to overcome academic and research practices' colonial and imperial legacies by promoting inclusivity, equity, and respect for indigenous knowledge and perspectives. While the specific principles may vary by context and discipline, the following are several principles commonly associated with decolonizing research methods (Smith, 2013; Thambinathan & Kinsella, 2021) and that, increasingly, we prioritize in our methods courses:

- **Acknowledging colonial histories**. Recognizing colonization's effects of on Indigenous peoples and their knowledge systems is crucial. Researchers must acknowledge colonialism's role in shaping existing research paradigms and marginalizing Indigenous knowledge.
- **Centering Indigenous knowledge**. Decolonizing research methods involves giving prominence to Indigenous knowledge, epistemologies, and ways of knowing. Researchers should respect and integrate Indigenous perspectives, practices, and worldviews.
- **Community participation and consent**. Prioritizing community involvement and obtaining informed consent are essential principles of decolonized research. Researchers should collaborate with Indigenous communities whenever relevant, part of which means seeking their approval and input throughout the research process.
- **Reflexivity and positionality**. Researchers should examine their own biases, assumptions, and positionalities in relation to their research topic and the communities they study. Such self-awareness helps address power imbalances and promote more equitable research relationships.
- **Empowerment and ownership**. Decolonizing research involves empowering Indigenous communities to take ownership of their knowledge and the research process. Researchers cannot exploit Indigenous knowledge for personal gain or academic recognition.
- **Ethical considerations**. Ethical frameworks must be culturally sensitive and adapted to community-specific values and norms. Researchers should consider the potential risks and benefits of their work and prioritize the well-being of the participants and the community.
- **Nonextractive research**. Research should not extract knowledge from Indigenous communities without either

reciprocating or contributing to those communities' well-being and development.

- **Diverse methodologies and epistemologies**. Embracing research methodologies and epistemologies beyond the dominant Western paradigms fosters a more inclusive and pluralistic research landscape.
- **Decolonizing data analysis and interpretation**. Data analysis and interpretation should avoid imposing Western-centric interpretations and not disregard Indigenous worldviews. Researchers should aim to present findings that reflect the perspectives of the communities they studied.
- **Engaging in ongoing dialogue and learning**. Decolonization is an ongoing, iterative process. Researchers ought to be open to learning from Indigenous communities and engage in ongoing critical discussions to improve their methods and practices.

The classroom is a critical space for beginning the process of decolonizing qualitative public health research methods. As we introduce students to qualitative studies, we allow ourselves to consider, together, whether a research plan is attentive enough to power dynamics or the broader shared history of researcher and subject. In having our students consider whether the power between the researcher and the researched acknowledges and is responsive to inequities that have historically been ignored by researchers, we encourage opportunities to rebalance power dynamics as an important criterion for their future projects.

Ethical consideration: The safety and well-being of the researcher

When we think about research ethics, our focus is usually on protecting study participants. To the extent that we go beyond this, it might be to consider the physical safety of the researcher or research team. For example, there may be a need to establish safety protocols for researchers working in unfamiliar locations, or in settings where potential physical risk is more likely than in everyday life.

Further, in recent discussions with students and team members conducting qualitative methods research, we've become more attentive to the fact that real-world research can create vulnerabilities and risks beyond physical safety. Qualitative research often means trying to experience the world as others do: we make space for people to share thoughts and experiences with issues and events that are meaningful to them. Doing so means giving up considerable control of what our research exposes us to. Thus, by its nature, qualitative research can be emotionally and physically taxing for the researcher.

Qualitative researchers may encounter the following:

- emotionally difficult encounters (e.g., interviews and/or observations)
- interviews that become difficult or upsetting
- problematic circumstances the research (or the researcher) does not have the capacity to address
- complex power dynamics between research institutions and historically marginalized communities

In higher-level courses and those that prepare students to enter the field, we set aside time to talk about the potential negative effects of some qualitative research on the emotional well-being of the researcher. You may find it valuable to have students discuss self-care and team care when it comes to difficult topics or challenging circumstances. It's good practice to be honest about what doing this research is like and to have your students think about how they can prepare for and deal with such challenges.

Rigor

We maintain that any qualitative methods course must engage with how to establish and assess rigor for qualitative studies. As LaDonna and colleagues note, "Evidentiary value depends not only on the rigor of the research process and the richness of data generated [during interviews] but also on how clearly and effectively investigators report their findings and demonstrate their contributions"

(LaDonna et al., 2021). Rigor is important if students are going to undertake their own studies and for facilitating a critical evaluation of qualitative work. Students should be prompted to think about what distinguishes a good qualitative study from a poor one. Among qualitative researchers, there has been considerable discussion of whether the same concepts used to assess qualitative studies are appropriate for considerations of rigor; you may want to center this debate in your course.

When we talk about a study's rigor, what we're asking is: "Why should someone believe this study's assertions?" or "What makes this study's findings useful for yielding data that can improve lives, policy, or practice?" Similarly, a class on rigor might start with straightforward questions like, "How and why would you feel confident using data generated in a study?" After posing these questions, you can have your students create their own foundation for considerations of rigor and compare their ideas with one or more approaches to qualitative rigor. Box 7.3 includes fundamental building blocks to help the students get started; Box 7.4 offers prompts that will aid you with this discussion.

Depending on the course's level, audience, and objectives, you may wish to present one or more sets of criteria for qualitative rigor. We generally start with concepts that students know from their training in quantitative research, such as validity (internal and external), reliability, and objectivity, and discuss how they do and don't apply to qualitative studies. Validity is not a term that is embraced by all qualitative researchers even though credibility concerns are universal (Peräkylä, 2016). We also bring up the important study concepts of quality, trustworthiness, and authenticity.

Lincoln and Guba's (1985) constructivist criteria for rigor can be an important touchstone when scrutinizing the determination of rigor for qualitative methods. Their criteria highlight scientific trustworthiness and are structured parallel to—rather than as distinct from—traditional scientific criteria, with a clear consideration of the ways that a straightforward application of the traditional scientific concepts is often not helpful.

In the table below (Table 7.1), we outline traditional scientific criteria alongside Lincoln and Guba's and provide questions that signify what is determined in a related assessment. This table can be a useful tool to present and discuss with students.

In advanced classes, or when you have more time to engage extensively with ideas of what makes a study rigorous, you might find it appropriate to also discuss Guba and Lincoln's later (1994) alternative criteria of Fairness, Evocation, and Critical Change. These concepts move somewhat beyond parallelism with the traditional criteria, embracing instead the importance of assessing the extent to which research is undertaken in partnership and has the potential for meaningful change. (We would however advise that with novice students or without sufficient time, these later criteria can be confusing, rather than clarifying.)

Another perspective on qualitative rigor is Daniel's (2018) Trustworthiness, Auditability, Credibility, and Transferability framework

Table 7.1 Lincoln and Guba's (1985) trustworthiness framework

Traditional scientific criteria	Trustworthiness parallel
Internal validity Did you find the truth?	**Credibility** Do the findings represent a believable interpretation of the data? Have you succeeded in capturing the phenomenon of interest?
External validity (generalizability) Do the findings hold outside of the study sample?	**Transferability** Is there applicability of knowledge derived from a study to other situations?
Reliability Could the study be repeated with the same results?	**Dependability** If someone audited your field notes, transcripts, and other study documents, would they conclude that your research process made sense?
Objectivity Is there enough "distance" to eliminate bias?	**Confirmability** Are the products (interpretations, conclusions, recommendations) of the research supported by the data collected? Is there relative freedom from unacknowledged biases?

(TACT). TACT is an effective tool for presenting concepts related to qualitative rigor in an educational setting. The TACT framework does not necessarily align with a specific epistemological or ontological stance on qualitative rigor, nor does it offer definitive rubrics for assessment. Rather, it is a straightforward approach to considerations of rigor that unites essential dimensions from the methodological literature. (See Table 7.2 for a description of TACT elements.)

Table 7.2 Daniel's (2018) TACT framework

TACT framework element	Components
Trustworthiness	audience confidence in the quality of the investigation demonstration of the integrity of process dependable outcomes findings situated in participant perspectives sources and quality of data researcher capacity and competence researcher's active engagement in reflexive practice
Auditability	transparency of data collection decisions documentation of research processes capacity for other researchers to follow and understand research processes systematic approach to data analysis data verification field notes and memos as audit tools
Credibility	establish findings as credible, relevant, and congruent anchoring analysis in participants' perspectives engagement in member checking use of theory in study design and approach description of data analysis and verification of data sources triangulation or convergence of data use of different data sources
Transferability	detailed description of phenomenon description of context delimitation of study acknowledgement of multiple realities accurate reflection of views of participants study description offers lessons for similar settings

Box 7.3 Qualitative building blocks: Strategies for building and demonstrating rigor

It is important for students to know various strategies that they can employ to build rigor into their studies. Below, we list several common study components that demonstrate a degree of rigor from a qualitative stance.

- **Prolonged engagement**. The more time you spend with a person or situation, the more insight you are likely to acquire.
- **Rich data** or **thick description**. There is often more value in depth than breadth in qualitative studies. There is also value in hearing what people say about things or having the specifics of a situation described. The devil is in the details—which is precisely where the insights are to be found.
- **Triangulation**. Coming at a problem from different angles will usually help build a fuller understanding of it. These angles can include data sources, methods or analysis, and theoretical approaches or investigators. Look for when different points reinforce one another; look also for when they show further differences. You will gain insight from including more than one contribution. And remember that not all data must agree for research to be of value.
- **Respondent validation** or **member checking**. Would the people in your study agree with your interpretation of the data? Would they recognize themselves in your presentation? These questions don't necessarily determine the utility of an analysis. Rather, they allow an assessment of the extent to which the researcher is connected to their participants' lives, which should shape how a reader assesses interpretation.
- **Negative cases**. Once you have an emerging idea of a phenomenon, it is often very valuable to look for examples of cases or data that do *not* fit your developing notion.

continued

Box 7.3 *continued*

- **External audit**. Can a colleague follow your process? Do they understand what you did and why you did it? Can they see how you came to interpret the data the way you did?

One challenge in teaching rigor in qualitative studies is where to place this content in the course. Putting it right at the beginning is a compelling thought; you could then use it to frame the rest of the course. But you may have an easier time getting your students to engage with concepts of rigor once they have a good sense of what qualitative methods are and how and with what purpose they are done. Students will need considerable qualitative familiarity before they can really understand why the traditional criteria for conceptualizing and assessing rigor may not be appropriate for qualitative research methods. We've introduced rigor both in the beginning and toward the end of our courses at different points in time. Ultimately, we don't have a strong recommendation for the best placement. We can say, though, that you should be prepared to consider rigor throughout the course in addition to the point at which you introduce it specifically.

Box 7.4 Tips and tricks: Using the Socratic method to engage students in what constitutes qualitative rigor

---

If you introduce methodological rigor near the end of a qualitative course, the Socratic method can help students teach each other by posing a series of questions for which they should have sufficient background to answer and formulate their own understanding. You will likely have already problematized the concept of objectivity earlier in the course. Getting students to recognize and articulate the applicability of specific criteria for determining study quality can in turn keep them from getting stuck on the idea that qualitative researchers claim assessments of rigor to be irrelevant.

> **Prompt 1**: In science, we are often told that internal validity—the extent to which observed results reflect truth without biases—is essential for a rigorous study. From what we've discussed in this course so far, does internal validity pose any challenges for qualitative research?
>
> **Prompt 2**: Let's turn to external validity—the idea that the conclusions of a scientific study can be applied to other contexts, situations, or populations. What issues does this raise for qualitative studies, given what we have learned about how good qualitative research is done?
>
> **Prompt 3**: Reliability is the idea that the scientific process should be repeatable: a researcher who repeats the work of another will generate the same results and reach the same conclusions. What do you think about reliability in relation to what we have covered in this course?

Regardless of when you teach rigor, make sure that all of your qualitative methods courses compel your students to think about distinguishing strong studies from weak ones. Qualitative methods are part of the scientific process. It is vital that students of qualitative methods have a good framework for assessing when work is done well and when it is not—just as it is vital that instructors prompt their students to consider the extent to which traditional concepts of rigor fit their understanding of how qualitative research is and should be done.

Reflexivity

In qualitative research, we often talk about the researcher as the instrument of data collection. Reflexivity is the examination of this fact—an interrogation of how various aspects of one's identity (see Box 7.5) shape the research conducted, the data generated, and the interpretation and utilization of findings. It's not too different from looking in the mirror before going to work to check how you will be presenting yourself (Figure 7.2).

An explicit embrace of reflexive practice can be one of the major differences between how qualitative researchers undertake research and how qualitative researchers typically conceptualize the scientific process. A reflexive researcher accounts for how they carry out their research and the ways that the person or team conducting the research influences that process.

To help your students engage with reflexivity, you might make the concept a priority in a guest lecture as part of a broader research discussion. In a qualitative course, the instructor will need to challenge the idea that objectivity is desirable or even possible in the conduct of research being outlined. You might also challenge objectivity as a plausible goal whether the research is qualitative or quantitative—but that goes beyond any expectations for a qualitative course! Generally, qualitative methods acknowledge and embrace reflexivity.

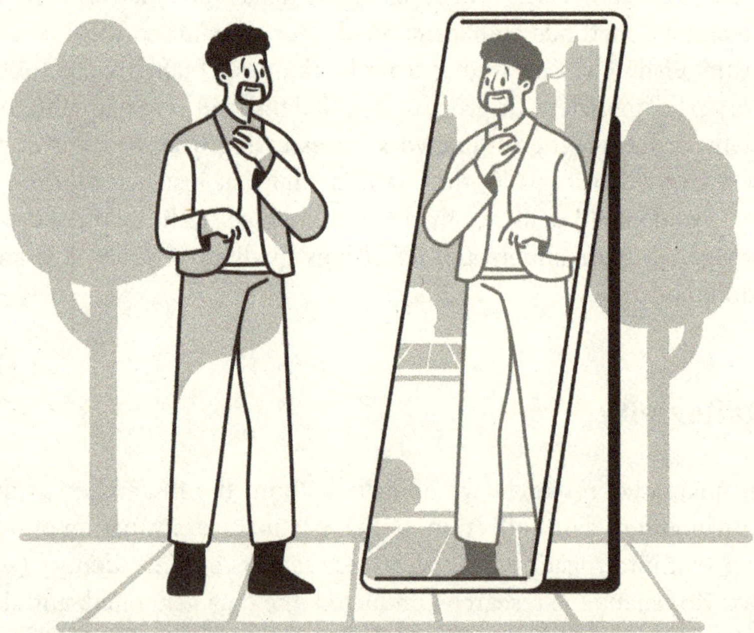

Figure 7.2 Reflexivity is a consideration of the impact of who the researcher is on the process undertaken and the data generated

Reflexive questions include the following:

- What is the context for the research?
- What are the questions? How and why were these prioritized?
- How are data being generated?
- How is the researcher interpreting their data?
- How are the research priorities and activities shaped by the researcher's identity?
- How do those priorities determine the focus and conduct of the research?
- How are people in the research setting being influenced by who is doing the research?
- How will interpretation of the findings of the research be shaped by who conducted it?

Reflexivity also means acknowledging that research is the product of situated human interaction (Box 7.5). While the researcher's characteristics are important, the subject of the research also shapes the interaction.

Box 7.5 Qualitative building blocks: Reflexivity considerations

---

Characteristics to consider relative to the factors that will likely shape the research process include the following:

- sociodemographic characteristics of the researcher and the study subject and participants
- historical, geographical, and political context of the research
- the researcher's theoretical background, professional training, and institutional affiliation
- the belief systems, personality, and lived experiences of the researcher and the participants

Students new to reflexivity can fixate on the idea that there is one set of identities or characteristics that make for the exact right person to undertake a particular research project. We encourage you to help students see how different people will be able to do different studies or do them in different ways. Insiders—those who come from an emic perspective—will learn different lessons from outsiders, or those who have etic perspectives. One is not inherently more valuable than the other—the value of each depends on the nature of the research question and the circumstances of the research. In all instances, the researcher must consider how their positionality shapes their process and the resulting data. Box 7.6 includes some ideas for engaging with students around the concept of reflexivity.

Box 7.6 Tips and tricks: Engaging students in reflexive practice

---

Exercise A

We routinely prompt our students with a public health topic and community or setting, such as the following:

- sleeping practices for families with children under one year old
- safety equipment for a given sport (e.g., skateboarding, dirt biking, mountain biking, horseback riding)
- self-concept among breast cancer survivors
- long-term medication adherence in a low-resource setting

We then ask students to spend a few minutes jotting down three to five ways in which aspects of their identity could shape the following:

- how they approach a given research topic and the questions they might prioritize
- how people perceive them and the research, and the responses they are likely to get

- the access they would be granted

Next, in pairs or small groups, we have our students discuss whether they all pointed to the same identity aspects and any implications of their own position or others on how a study might be undertaken.

You can revisit this exercise near the end of the course, when students have a better understanding of methods and have thought more about collecting data (or even practiced doing so). The exercise is a good introduction to reflexivity.

Exercise B

In more practice-based classes, where students are undertaking a real-world qualitative project, we have them write a Researcher Identity Memo, as described by Maxwell (2005). Maxwell has encouraged researchers to write a memo examining "your goals, experiences, assumptions, feelings, and values as they relate to your research, and to discover what resources and potential concerns your identity and experience may create." The researcher is encouraged not to write a general account of their goals, background, and experiences, but instead to describe specifically those that are most relevant to their research project. When doing this exercise, we first encourage students to brainstorm their goals, background, and experiences as they relate to the research project at hand. We then ask them to reflect on how these may create advantages, or disadvantages, for their study.

In advanced classes, you might take this exercise one step further by presenting the concept of the Three Selves:

- **Research-based self**: who are we in relation to the specific research project? What do we bring to this research endeavor?
- **Brought self**: who are we—what are our historic and social contexts and our individual standpoints. What do we bring with us wherever we go?
- **Situationally created self**: what about us shapes our interactions with research participants in this specific project?

continued

> **Box 7.6** *continued*
>
> ---
>
> This practice may be best approached as an individual writing exercise in response to a research prompt. Reflexivity practices are, appropriately, both personal and public. Offering students a personal reflexive exercise, read only by their instructor, may result in greater engagement and vulnerability throughout the course.
>
> Demonstrating these practices to students also allows you to discuss how sharing reflexive practices can build research trustworthiness. We have had faculty prepare and present considerations of self as they relate to their own work before assigning our classes a written Researcher Identity Memo or Three Selves Activity.

Reflexive practice requires us to interrogate how each of our selves influences our research efforts, as those efforts are shaped by and staged around the binaries, contradictions, and paradoxes of our own lives. As reflexive researchers, we reflect upon how we shape our identities in the field, in the writing process, in interactions with respondents—in all presentations of our work.

Summary

This chapter underscores the essential integration of ethics and rigor throughout qualitative research courses and emphasizes the multifaceted considerations beyond traditional methods. Ethical dimensions—including informed consent within iterative designs and ensuring anonymity while maintaining data richness—are paramount. Reflexivity emerges as a pivotal concept, challenging notions of objectivity and leading students to a self-examination of their roles in the research process. Teaching rigor is a nuanced challenge, one complicated by the question of when in the curriculum to introduce it. By embracing reflexivity alongside ethical and rigorous practices, students will be equipped with the foundational skills they need to navigate the complexities of qualitative research responsibly and effectively.

8

Teaching Writing and Dissemination of Qualitative Studies

If you are teaching a course in which advanced students will write up their own qualitative research studies, you'll want to consider how you provide guidance on qualitative-research-related writing. The first book in this series, Jennifer Beard's *Teaching Public Health Writing* (2022), is a great resource for anyone embarking on a course in which writing is a central component. We assume that most qualitative methods courses won't include a significant amount of writing- and dissemination-related content, but most courses would likely benefit from some engagement with the effective dissemination of qualitative work.

Teaching qualitative research dissemination and maximizing impact

Before starting the write-up and dissemination of any study results, it's helpful to ask a few questions about goals and audience, including the following:

- What question(s) do I want to answer?
- What aspects of my data do I want to focus on?
- Who is the audience (e.g., policymakers, participants, stakeholders, academics)?

Teaching Qualitative Research in Public Health. Katherine Clegg Smith et al., Oxford University Press.
© Oxford University Press (2026). DOI: 10.1093/9780197662472.003.0008

- How can I reach that audience?
- How do I want to present my findings (e.g., descriptive, theoretically engaged, action-oriented)?

Your answers will determine the dissemination venue, influence the format of your presentation, and may help inform who is involved in writing up and communicating the findings. Some people may want to spend hours crafting a 3,000-word manuscript for peer review, while others may prioritize the preparation of research briefs for advocacy purposes or explaining the implications of the research findings for local legislators, and still others may need to write a short memo for their supervisor at the health department.

In our experience, public health courses often neglect the process of writing, publishing, and disseminating; instead, students tend to learn this process through an apprenticeship-type model. Rarely are public health students explicitly trained to present research effectively—that is, in a way that policymakers and other practitioners find meaningful. Students are often taught far more skills in doing research than in communicating their findings to audiences who can use and build upon them. There is arguably a more pressing need to ensure that students trained in qualitative methods are prepared to share their work, as these students are more likely to encounter a peer or a mentor with quantitative methods experience and may be alone at their worksite in their command of qualitative research methods. Unfortunately, this communication skill gap can gravely limit the potential impact of the work. Qualitative work that never gets disseminated can never help improve public health.

Dissemination can include a range of formats specific to academic and nonacademic audiences. However, we acknowledge that it is difficult—if not impossible—to provide a precise recipe for writing up a good qualitative paper. Beyond the written product, your students may need guidance on how to disseminate their work, whether in peer-reviewed journals, white papers, reports, and memos, or on the internet and social media.

Publishing peer-reviewed literature: Writing for an academic audience

As a qualitative course instructor, you will likely spend most of your class time on the foundational skills necessary for engaging with and thinking about qualitative data, and you may find it difficult to separate writing from analysis. Should you include a limited unit on writing or disseminating qualitative research, you run the risk of treating writing as a discrete stage in the research process. Indeed, the research process for quantitative studies is regularly presented as one in which data collection and analytic work are followed by the straightforward "writing up" of findings.

This linearity, though, is atypical, as is the idea that writing is a separate activity from analysis (see Chapter 6). Richardson (2005), in *Writing: A Method of Inquiry*, observes, "I write because I want to find something out. I write in order to learn something that I did not know before I wrote it." From this perspective, writing is a method of discovery and analysis: a creative process, rather than a mechanistic activity that occurs after the researcher knows what the story is. Similarly, Timmermans and Tavory (2022, p. 134) have reminded us that

> analysis resides in the writing itself. Writing is not a mop-up chore at the end of a research project. To write is to make countless choices of what pieces of evidence to present; what metaphors are most convincing; whose narrative voice to use; whether to develop a scene, a setting, a concept, or a theme; and what transformations in your main characters will carry a theoretical arc.

At the same time, courses dedicated to scientific writing with the goal of preparing students to write manuscripts for peer review may be framed around the write-up of quantitative study results. In our experience, quantitative research papers tend to be much more standardized across journals and disciplines than qualitative peer-reviewed articles in terms of content and format. Pratt (2009) suggested that qualitative work *must* do the following:

- honor the participants' worldview
- provide sufficient evidence for the claims it makes
- contribute to theory

And qualitative work *should* do the following:

- show more than tell
- go beyond description
- resist imposing quantitative philosophy and concepts

Pratt's principles expect that a detailed account will center the qualitative data itself and make connections to earlier and future investigations (via theory). They have called on qualitative researchers to disseminate while avoiding reductionism and quantification.

The typical word limit for public health and clinical journals (3,000–4,000 words) can be a challenge for publishing qualitative research, given the need to include often lengthy quotes as data. Embrace this challenge: present your class with the dilemma of balancing their need to demonstrate the data upon which they draw their conclusions with the brevity required by so many journals.

We have the following three goals when teaching writing for an academic audience:

1. Expose students to the diversity of formats and styles for qualitative research articles.
2. Develop students' ability to incorporate data into their manuscripts.
3. Prepare students to describe their methodological approach and analysis process consistent with a qualitative epistemological paradigm.

Goal #1: Understanding the diversity of article styles and formats

Student engagement with qualitative texts will usually vary. There is a chance that some of your students may have never read a qualitative research article, let alone a full monograph based on qualitative research, such as an ethnography. Some may have a very narrow sense of what a research article should look like, what the tone and style should be, what should be included, and how it should be structured. Unfortunately, this schema usually represents writing standards for quantitative research and does not reflect the diversity of formats and styles found in qualitative peer-reviewed articles. Such diversity can often confuse students, and the lack of a standard format—i.e., how to use data, how and where to use theory, how to use quotes, and the balance among data, theory, and interpretation—can overwhelm them.

To account for this, we will compile a series of publications from several journals that represent the general range of qualitative peer-reviewed articles. You may want to choose some articles from public health or medical journals, and some articles from journals oriented to other disciplines (e.g., anthropology, sociology), and representing the range of public health content. Depending on the size of your class, you may want to be intentional about selecting articles that reflect your students' interests. To further highlight the differences in format, content, and style, you may find it helpful to identify multiple articles on the same topic, or by the same author(s).

In preparation for an in-class activity, a take-home assignment with a reflective essay, or a series of interactive online discussion forum posts, ask your students to select and read two or three of the articles from the list provided and consider the following 10 questions:

- How do the authors use theory?
- Do the authors include a positionality statement?

- Where are the findings interpreted (e.g., are interpretations woven throughout the text, or are they only in the discussion section)?
- Where is the description of the study population or the data that inform the results?
- How do the authors describe their methods—at what level of detail? How do they describe specific aspects of the study, such as sampling or data analysis?
- What markers of rigor or quality do you see in each article?
- How do the selection and presentation of data vary between research articles for specialized academic communities and those written for a more general audience?
- How do differences in data presentation impact the analytical depth and the complexity of the arguments being made?
- What are the main findings the authors present?
- How do the qualities discussed in response to the prior questions shape your assessment of the findings?

Having students engage with the form and style of multiple articles after reading several articles can help them understand the choices that published authors make and the choices they will make about how to present their own studies, the audiences they want to write for—and the consequences of these choices. For example, a qualitative article in a journal with a 3,000-word limit will communicate something very different than a 10,000-word article and will do so for a very different readership. For those students who are pursuing practice-oriented careers, such exercises will strengthen their analytic skills and enhance their ability to effectively translate qualitative papers for their work settings.

Goal #2: Incorporating data into manuscripts

Traditionally, qualitative research is written in such a way that data extracts (quotes) are interspersed with the author's analytic presentation. This approach is essentially incompatible with the

3,000–4,000 word limit for many journals—unless the scope of the paper is extremely limited. One adaptive strategy for qualitative researchers publishing in clinical and public health outlets has been to move data extracts to a table/tables that are then referenced in the text. When deciding whether to include quotes in the text or in a table, students will need to consider the balance between readability, coherence, and the significance of the information. External considerations include the context in which the research will be presented (e.g., does the target journal have a standard practice?) and the quotes' clarity—whether readers will need an explanatory narrative to make sense of them.

You can begin your students' consideration by discussing the significance of quotes for supporting arguments and providing evidence. When the quotes contribute to narrative flow or emphasize key points, students may want to integrate them straight into the text. However, when dealing with numerous quotes or detailed data that might clutter the text, tables can help them present their information in a concise and organized manner. Putting quotes in tables can also be highly practical: some journals' word limits do not include tables. With that said, readability and aesthetics may require tabled quotes to be shorter than they would be if integrated into the text. Further, data in tables are inevitably separated from textual interpretation, meaning the writer must take extra care to ensure that the data illuminate points in the text.

We find the "excerpt strategy" articulated by Emerson, Fretz, and Shaw (2011, pp. 215–216) a particularly helpful model for incorporating quotes and other data into the main text. This strategy has the author begin with an *analytic point* that contributes to the theme of the section or overall paper. Following the analytic point, the author provides *orienting information*: information that bridges the analytic point and the illustrative excerpt. This information can include the participant's demographic characteristics, profession/role, or other background information relevant to the topic or that helps the reader interpret the quote or data that follows. After the orienting information comes the *excerpt* (e.g., quote, field note); after the excerpt, the author writes an *analytic commentary*, highlighting the issues that the data excerpt raises and connecting them to broader themes or analytic insights so the reader can identify the excerpt's takeaways.

We also use this part of the class to discuss editing quotes for reader comprehension. We emphasize that decisions about how to represent participants on the page carry political implications and are not purely neutral, technical tasks. As such, the process of incorporating quotes should be disclosed in the description of methods so that readers are aware of the decisions made and can read and interpret the findings with full knowledge of how the author approached the incorporation of quotes into the written product before them. The chosen transcription conventions, including punctuation, formatting, and even word choice, carry biases and reflect and recreate power dynamics. Whether it's the selection of depiction of dialects and accents in quoted speech, the decision to include or omit non-verbal cues like pauses or emphases, or the position of speech attributions, each choice reflects underlying societal norms, linguistic hierarchies, and cultural prejudices and should also be detailed in methods sections. Thus, your students' editorial decisions influence not only the readability and accuracy of the text but their audience's perceptions, and they can reinforce or challenge existing power structures. In our more advanced classes, we usually embed this discussion within a larger conversation about how speech is represented on the page and the considerations that come with "cleaning it up"—that is, the often-hidden assumptions about race, class, gender, immigration status, and education that undergird such judgments. Box 8.1 offers an example from one of our studies on how to incorporate teaching about the use of quotes into your course.

Box 8.1 Tips and tricks: Using and editing quotes

Students might be unaware of exactly how to incorporate quotes into text (for example, by writing around quotes, guiding the reader to the analytic insight in the quote); how to provide enough context to interpret the speaker's words; how to edit quotes for comprehension for readers unfamiliar with the data whence the quotes come; and how to use quotes strategically given restrictive page and word limits. One exercise that helps students develop a sense of the different ways they can use data involves giving them a series of writing scenarios based on data excerpts of varying length and complexity. In the following example, we would provide students with quotes from a particular code from a transcript. In our example, we use a recently completed study led by Owczarzak and Smith on living with Multiple Sclerosis (MS).

Example #1: Interview excerpt with information in multiple places in narrative

Identify a transcript excerpt in which a participant's response to a question spreads across several sections of a transcript, for example, a story that contains essential information at the beginning and the end but is interrupted by information that is not relevant to the analytic point you are making within the text. Provide students with a prompt about using the quote, such as, "You want to use this participant's experience to describe how people with severe MS engage in everyday activities. Which parts of the quote will you use? How would you edit them to create one coherent narrative?"

Example #2: Lengthy, detailed excerpt

Identify a transcript excerpt in which a participant tells a very long, detailed, and rich story that captures a fundamental or unique experience. Tell students that they should imagine that they are preparing a manuscript with a 3,500-word limit, and they will have to edit the quote or paraphrase the story for the publication. Ask them to identify the essential elements of the quote to illustrate the experience and how they would tailor it and the story to fit within the word limit.

Example #3: Practice "writing around" quotes

Identify a succinct, clear quote from the data that illustrates a central experience or key insight into the data. Ask students to practice the

continued

> **Box 8.1** *continued*
>
> ---
>
> "excerpt strategy" in which they introduce the participant's quote, present the quote and information about the participant, and summarize the key insight that emerges from it.

Goal #3: Describing methods and analysis

A persistent problem with writing up qualitative studies is the amount of detail to include in the methods section—particularly the description of data analysis. It's likewise important to understand whether to describe generic processes (e.g., "We developed a code system") or a study-specific process (e.g., "Authors JO and KS read the transcript independent of each other and identified preliminary topics, such as provider experience and training and ideas about drug use"). We encourage students to identify journals in which they'd like to publish and study the structure, style, and content of qualitative papers those journals have published. Depending on the word limit, there might only be room for a few short paragraphs on data collection and analysis. We've also found it useful to include writing exercises as part of our courses. Box 8.2 offers an example of how to do that.

Following Saldaña (2015), we recommend students include the following:

- a description of the study participants and data collected
- references to the literature that guided their analysis
- how they organized and managed the data (e.g., whether they used software; when and where they translated)
- their code-developing process (who was involved; whether they used an inductive or deductive approach)
- how the process of coding the data unfolded
- the process of data analysis after coding

The last item in this list seems to be particularly difficult for students because it requires them to make explicit some of the subconscious categorization at the core of qualitative data analysis and theory-building (Grodal et al., 2021). Often, journal articles mention this step only briefly, if they mention it at all.

Box 8.2 Tips and tricks: Writing about qualitative methods and analysis

To help students practice this type of writing, we use two versions of an assignment. The first asks them to write a plan of analysis for data that will be collected; the second has them summarize data they already analyzed. We tell students to include the following elements in each write-up:

- a brief description of the data set
- the purpose of the data collection
- sample characteristics
- types of data
- the number of observations or interviews
- the data set's strengths and limitations
- a research question you would/did try to answer with the data
- the study's focus (breadth or depth)
- the unit of analysis (e.g., individual, couple, group, organization, community, system)
- a description of how they answered (or would answer) the research question with the available data
- how they will establish coding reliability, including reconciling discrepancies
- which between-group comparisons they will make, if any, and how they will do so
- how they will account for new and unanticipated findings in their analysis

Related to the description of methods and analysis is the question of study limitations. It is a personal pet peeve for us when the first line of the limitations section for a qualitative paper is some variation of, "This study is limited due to the small sample size." Not at all: a small sample size is almost always appropriate for a qualitative study! Indeed, the capacity to undertake in-depth analysis due to a focused sample is often a *strength* of qualitative research. Instead of being bashful about the supposed limitations of a qualitative approach, make your limitations section study-specific.

We teach our students to reflect on their studies' limitations by reconsidering one or more of each study's elements, including the following:

- **Methodological limitations**. These include shortcomings in the research design, such as sampling methods, data collection techniques, or analysis procedures.
- **Sampling issues**. Such issues are limitations of the sample diversity or representativeness of the participants *vis-a-vis* the topic at hand, and not in terms of generalizability (which is not the goal of a qualitative approach).
- **Data collection challenges**. Among these difficulties are participant engagement, data quality, and the researcher's role.
- **Analytic constraints**. Limitations of the data analysis process include the process of developing codes, coding consensus and application, and challenges synthesizing or incorporating diverse perspectives into the analysis and interpretation of findings.
- **Contextual constraints**. External factors or contextual influences such as time constraints and resource availability may have affected the research or the findings.
- **Consideration of transferability**. Acknowledge the potential limitations of the study's applicability beyond its context or sample population and discuss the extent to which its findings may be transferable to other settings or populations.

Finally, it is increasingly common for journals to ask authors to include a positionality statement. These statements offer readers insight into the researcher's background and potential influence on the study's design, data collection, analysis, and interpretation. By asking potential authors to acknowledge their own subjectivity and its possible effect on their findings, journals aim to improve the credibility and trustworthiness of the research they publish. Additionally, by highlighting the diverse perspectives and experiences that shape research outcomes, positionality statements can foster a more inclusive, reflective scholarly community.

Whether positionality statements have this effect is an open question. As Robertson (2002) observed, the experiences and aspects of identity that these statements include are often "generic, fixed categories" and "ready to wear identities" that can preclude deeper reflections on power, authority, and voice in the research process (p. 789). To help ready your students for this aspect of writing about qualitative research findings, and hopefully engage in the deeper reflections Robertson laments, consider the exercise we describe in Box 8.3.

Box 8.3 Tips and tricks: Positionality statements

Leading a guided reflection on positionality is one strategy for helping your students think through their approach to such statements.

1. **Introduction**. Provide an overview of positionality and the purpose of positionality statements.
   - Present positionality statements from published papers.
   - As a class, analyze their structure and content.
   - Discuss the students' own reactions to these statements. How revealing are the statements? How do they help the students understand the research process and the authors' role in it?

continued

Box 8.3 *continued*

---

2. **Guided reflection**. Ask the students to reflect on their own positionality.
   - What personal experiences, beliefs, and biases might influence your research?
   - How might your social, cultural, or professional background shape your perspective?
   - What potential power dynamics exist between you and your participants?
   - How do you navigate your role as a researcher within the research process?
3. **Small group discussion**. Reflect on the guiding questions.
   - Divide the students into small groups for discussion of their guided reflections.
4. **Write a positionality statement**. Based on the guided reflection and small group discussion, have the students draft their own positionality statements.
   - Pair students to exchange drafts of their positionality statements.
   - Ask students to provide constructive feedback on clarity, depth of reflection, and areas for improvement.

Considering language and culture

Language and culture issues are often at the heart of qualitative methods and analysis and require us to confront questions of power, legitimacy, voice, and authority. We recommend engaging with these topics at several different points during each qualitative course.

As we discussed above, transcription is a powerful tool and thus an excellent place to talk about language and culture. Even if your intent is to transcribe verbatim, the word-for-word translation of spoken words into written text requires countless decisions about language and representation. How should you render dialect? If a participant speaks in slang, should you "clean up" their language to standardize it for your audience? Should you include curse words, or censor them? Should your quotations include "um" and incorrect grammar? Box 8.4 includes an example of how different translations can be and provides a concrete reference for classroom discussions.

Having your students practice transcription in class and then compare their results is an invaluable exercise for helping them understand the implications of their decisions on how we interpret participants' experiences—and therefore how important these decisions are. To find appropriate audio, you might visit one of the following sources:

- personal narratives about health, such as those collected by the Health Experience Research Network (HERN) (https://www.healthexperiencesusa.org)
- oral history collections at the National Archives (https://www.archives.gov/about/history/oral-history-at-the-national-archives)
- life history projects, such as the Chincoteague Island Life History Project (https://chincoteaguemuseum.com/life-history/)

After you've chosen and played your audio, you might want to ask some or all of the following questions:

- To what extent does your transcript capture participant-interviewer interactions?
- How did you decide whether to include pauses, "um," stops and starts, and the like?
- Are there instances where you wanted to clean up the speech to make it more understandable as written text?
- If transcribing from video: to what extent did you include nonverbal elements of communication in the transcript?
- What decisions did you make about punctuation, such as when to use dashes and ellipses?

These issues of language and culture can arise much earlier in the research process—for example, when the primary spoken language (or the only one) is different from that of the researcher. Language differences can arise between researchers fluent in different languages, researchers and study participants, and researchers and an audience, as with the dissemination of findings through English-language peer-reviewed publications. When language differences are present, explaining your translation decisions and processes becomes even more important. Here are a few questions to consider.

- What materials did you translate (e.g., protocols, data collection instruments, field notes, analytic products, reports)?
- Who translated? Did one person translate all material and a second person check for accuracy? Did you need multiple translations? Did you back-translate into the source language? Who resolved the discrepancies?
- What specific skills did the translator have? For example, if your work involves a unique vocabulary, your translator needs to be proficient in both the source and target languages.
- When did you translate—immediately after the interview, or after working in the source language as much as possible for as long as possible, translating key concepts and categories after you'd reached the analytical and dissemination process?

Box 8.4 Tips and tricks: Comparing translations

Sharing examples of the same text translated by different people can help emphasize the importance of language and translation in qualitative research. (You may well have plenty of examples from your own work; we share one example below.) The comparison can be the foundation for a class discussion on translation issues as outlined above.

"Our organization has worked with 2 different target groups, sex workers and people who inject drugs, and [we] determine in which group [the women] should be included based on her main risk-taking behavior (so-called 'leading' activities). These groups usually do not intersect with each other. For this project we have recruited only those women who inject drugs who are eligible for our HIV-prevention intervention; some of them had or have experience in providing commercial sex (for money, shelter, drugs, gifts …), and some of them have not. However, we also have clients who do not consider themselves sex workers, since they consider sex with several partners as friendly relationships (for mutual pleasure) and not a business. So, if their friends give them drugs, gifts, etc, it is a sign of good-will or a friendly gesture showing a good attitude toward her. Having a permanent sexual partner or husband at the same time does not change anything. It is very difficult psychologically for them to accept that they are sex workers. They have even demonstrated aggression and aversion toward sex workers."

"Our project has two different directions with the target groups of sex workers and IDUs […], which don't overlap between themselves. During our pilot [project], […] we invite[d] only the women who inject drugs eligible for our HIV prevention/ intervention [program], some of them have or had experiences of providing sex on the commercial basis (money, shelter, drugs, gifts.), and others don't. But there is also this group [of people], who doesn't consider them sex workers, explaining sex with multiple partners as friendly (for mutual pleasure). So if she received something for this (such as drugs, gifts, and etc.), it is a treat, a sign of goodwill or friendly gesture for a good relationship. Having a constant sex partner or husband does not change anything. Psychologically it is very difficult for them to accept and call themselves as sex workers. They even show aggression and contempt toward [the representatives of] this group [sex workers]."

More broadly, these questions of language and culture invite a consideration of the extent to which a site's culture and history should factor into preparation for fieldwork and data analysis. Such matters are relevant considerations for one's own country or community, as well as for communities where researchers are guests. Qualitative research prioritizes context in textual analysis, including social context (e.g., demographic characteristics, broader social forces), individual experiences (e.g., specifics and particulars of a person's life, social interactions), and the context of the research encounter (e.g., how questions are asked, interactional sequences). A site's cultural and historical intricacies shape its social dynamics, community interactions, and environmental relationships. Ignoring these factors can lead to misunderstandings, misinterpretations, and even conflicts during fieldwork. See Box 8.5 for consideration of colonization in the context of language and qualitative research.

Moreover, without a comprehensive understanding of culture and history, researchers risk overlooking critical insights and phenomena that may influence their analysis. Incorporating this understanding enriches the research process while fostering respect for the communities involved—and is consistent with ethical research practice. While teaching about specific cultural and historical contexts within a qualitative methods class is unrealistic and impractical, recognition of such issues can be undertaken in alignment with a consideration of emic and etic perspectives. Emic perspectives focus on understanding behavior and phenomena from *within* the culture being studied and emphasize insider perspectives, meanings, and interpretations. By contrast, etic perspectives prioritize an *external* viewpoint, analyzing phenomena through universal principles and concepts and often minimizing the specific cultural context.

The benefits of the emic perspective lie in its ability to provide rich, culturally sensitive insights and a deeper understanding of the studied culture. However, this perspective may lead to difficulty with cross-cultural comparison and generalization. Conversely, etic perspectives offer broader, comparative insights and facilitate the development of universal theories, yet risk oversimplifying cultural complexities and overlooking the nuances of specific contexts.

When discussing the perspectives in class, you might consider the following:

- what emic and etic perspectives can contribute to an understanding of health disparities

- how to integrate emic and etic perspectives into public health research to enhance an intervention's design and implementation
- how to incorporate emic and etic perspectives into research: who to include in projects, in what roles, and with what skills and expertise
- the ethical considerations of incorporating multiple perspectives into public health research and practice
- how to understand and take into account the evolving, contextual nature of identity

Emic and etic perspectives also provide an opportunity to discuss reflexivity and positionality, which we address in detail in Chapter 7.

Box 8.5 Qualitative building blocks: Language, dissemination, and decolonization

---

The English language's dominance in scientific literature is a longstanding issue that raises concerns about equity, diversity, and academic inclusion. The dominance of English creates barriers for researchers and knowledge producers who speak other languages, limiting their ability to access and contribute to global scientific discourse. Decolonization efforts in academia aim to address these imbalances by advocating for linguistic diversity, promoting the recognition and inclusion of Indigenous and local knowledge, and creating spaces for marginalized voices to be heard and valued within scientific communities. Initiatives such as translating research findings into multiple languages, supporting multilingual publications, and prioritizing Indigenous research methodologies are gaining traction as part of the broader decolonization of scientific literature.

Recognizing linguistic diversity within research teams can promote inclusivity in academic writing, in turn allowing for a more inclusive approach to writing. By including team members proficient in different

continued

> **Box 8.5** *continued*
>
> ---
>
> languages, researchers can include diverse perspectives and voices in scholarly discourse. This practice can improve accessibility for non-English speakers and result in a more equitable and inclusive research environment.

Publishing for an applied or nonacademic audience

Public health is an applied field. When training future generations of researchers, teaching students how to reach diverse audiences and maximize the impact of our work can help them realize the many ways to practice impactful science throughout their careers. Public health professionals work in clinical, community, and policy spaces across the world. Our work has implications for how health care is delivered; how interventions are fielded; how diseases and injuries and their treatments are understood; how policies are formulated, implemented, and enforced; and how all these efforts can be understood and evaluated. Impact, for us, has implications for scholarship, how care and services are provided, and how practitioners and policymakers understand the people they serve and how they can best promote the public's health. Ensuring students are equipped to tailor qualitative findings to the varied audiences they want to access their work is a worthy teaching objective.

Our approach to teaching how to disseminate qualitative research "outside of the ivory tower" is often a study in contrast. Writing for nonacademic audiences requires a different approach than writing for an academic audience. We began this chapter by highlighting key concepts to convey when teaching about publishing qualitative research. We approach teaching about writing for nonacademic audiences in the same way and invite you to consider the contrast between the two purposes and whether that contrast provides a useful framework for your classroom.

We've adapted Pratt's list of "musts" and "shoulds" to reflect our own set of rules for writing for nonacademic audiences. When writing for a nonacademic audience, qualitative work *must* do the following:

- consider the audience
- convey a small number of clear findings
- articulate the implications of those findings

And qualitative work *should* do the following:

- include examples (or stories) of people's experiences that bring the data to life
- be accessible
- invite feedback and input from people from the communities you want to reach

For nonacademic audiences, you must know who you are writing for and how to effectively reach them with a clear set of findings and implications that align with their needs and goals. Knowing your audience informs which research findings to highlight and how those findings are communicated.

Knowing your audience involves the following important considerations:

- What are the goals and priorities of your audience? What do they care about? How does that relate to your work?
- What level of knowledge do they have about qualitative research? About research in general?
- What level of knowledge do they have about the health topic or technical issues being addressed? What is their level of health literacy?
- How much time do they have to engage with your work? What format do they prefer to receive results? What length of document or style of presentation would be most appropriate?

- To what extent does your audience prioritize research and data versus stories and lived experiences?

Understanding the needs of a nonacademic audience can be challenging for some students. In particular, early career students may have limited experience working with different communities and less appreciation for how communication strategies can vary depending on who you are trying to reach. In such instances, we suggest using detailed vignettes that offer authentic learning experiences by asking students to identify a central message from an article and then creatively plan for how to convey that message and the supporting results in different styles—you might consider a one-page legislative memo for a policymaker's office, oral testimony as part of a legislative committee hearing, or a structured report for a funding agency. Vignettes can illustrate the need to approach the writing task differently when a reader is unlikely to engage in the same way as a reader of a peer-reviewed article.

One important issue is the possibility that a nonacademic audience will have more limited health literacy. Encouraging students to incorporate principles of health literacy into assignments that mimic writing for practitioners can help to routinize that practice. Take a guide, like the U.S. Centers for Disease Control and Prevention's Plain Language Checklist (CDC, 2023), and have students review written documents to see how well they adhere to the items on the checklist.

The style of writing for nonacademic audiences is also generally different. Practitioners and lay audiences often have limited time to engage with research findings. It is therefore best practice to put the most important messages first, break text up with headings and bullet points, and keep things simple. These practices are important in retaining the reader's attention. As a class exercise, you could give students a peer-reviewed article and ask them to rewrite the results using some of these techniques.

Writing for policymakers

Policies affect the public's health. Qualitative research findings can be incorporated into materials designed to educate policymakers and advocate for specific actions. Effective communication with policymakers tends to be brief; policymakers (and their staff) have limited time to spend on any one topic, so one-page memos and materials are standard. It is often appropriate to lead with clear and solutions-oriented asks, and to provide clear justification for that ask through the presentation of your work. The ability to situate public health "asks" within the communities that policymakers serve and the lives of real people is critical. Qualitative findings can provide the context and connection to the public that makes for powerful, persuasive communication with policymakers. Stories of individuals, rich descriptions of public health challenges, and the promise of policy solutions to address identified problems can resonate with and move policymakers to action. Incorporating policy communication skills into qualitative courses provides students with an additional skill set, offers an example of the variety of applications for qualitative findings, and invites students who are seeking nonacademic careers to consider how the method matters for their work.

Summary

Writing and dissemination are critical in getting qualitative public health research into the hands of those who can use it. Effective communication involves knowing your audience and sharing your findings in a way they can understand and appreciate. Exposing students to a range of writing styles, for both academic and nonacademic audiences, and asking them to practice developing materials for these different groups will help them to become effective public health messengers.

9

Evaluation of Understanding and Mastery of Key Concepts

Evaluating students' comprehension and mastery of qualitative concepts and skills can be quite a challenge because the indicators of good qualitative work seem so often to boil down to that old standby: "I know it when I see it." Moreover, rubrics and point values may seem antithetical to a qualitative mindset. Regardless, there are many good reasons to consider the best way to assess whether (and how) students grasp a course's key concepts, whether they can apply this knowledge to other scenarios, and whether they can think critically about the course content. But beyond these evaluation goals, assessment activities are also vital for determining whether a course is meeting its objectives and how it might be improved.

Considerations in developing assessments

We adopt a goal-centered approach to designing assessment methods. The assessment's goal should do the following:

- reflect the course's learning objectives
- draw upon the principles of authentic assessment whenever possible
- be consistent with the instructional team's grading capacity
- help students learn and understand themselves as future consumers and producers of qualitative research

Teaching Qualitative Research in Public Health. Katherine Clegg Smith et al., Oxford University Press.
© Oxford University Press (2026). DOI: 10.1093/9780197662472.003.0009

In addition to the following information and examples, we encourage you to seek the guidance of your institution's instructional design and pedagogy experts, or of any other resources you trust for pedagogical guidance.

Learning objectives

In Chapter 2, we discussed Backward Design in the context of course construction. Backward Design is also a key element in designing learner- and course-appropriate evaluations. In centering the idea that learning is a consecutive process, Bloom's Taxonomy classifies learning stages from remembering facts to creating new ideas based on acquired knowledge. It also functions as a framework for assessing and measuring the cognitive growth and development of learners as they progress from basic knowledge acquisition to higher-order thinking skills. In this way, instructors can use Bloom's Taxonomy to consider what they want students to learn in particular class sessions and at particular stages of their training, and to further determine their students' preparation for engagement with qualitative research after they've completed a course.

You can also use Bloom's Taxonomy to identify a course's learning objectives, determine the assessment evidence necessary to confirm that each objective has been met, and plan a learning experience to build that knowledge with students. For example, an instructor might expect students in a foundational qualitative methods course to have basic knowledge, such as how to read the methods and results of a peer-reviewed qualitative research paper. They probably would not expect them to have more sophisticated knowledge, such as the ability to design a qualitative research project. In contrast, an instructor of an advanced course may well expect students to design a qualitative study and provide a rationale for their sampling strategy and research questions.

Effective assessment of student learning should be grounded in clear objectives for the course and its components. By using your syllabus to outline the knowledge and skills you expect your students to acquire via the course and why these elements are important (and by repeating your explanation elsewhere as needed), you'll be well positioned to develop assessments that align with your learning objectives and course content. This alignment will also give your students a firm basis for their expectations about their own learning.

As instructors in a school of public health, we must also account for the Council on Education for Public Health's (CEPH) framework for assessing the quality of public health education. As of this writing, our context is the 2016 revisions, with an emphasis on ensuring alignment among course objectives, program competencies, learning outcomes, and assessments. CEPH review and accreditation assess whether each course or program of study learning objective has a specific place within the course content that conveys its "didactic opportunity" and a discrete, identifiable *individual* evaluation of that learning. For example, an example of a CEPH-aligned competency, content, and assessment for a foundational competency related to qualitative research looks like this:

Competency: 3b. Explain the role of qualitative methods and sciences in describing and assessing a population's health.

Didactic opportunity: Concepts in Qualitative Research for Social and Behavioral Sciences

Assessment opportunity: Assignment 3: An individual written assignment that covers: 1) selecting a health-related question and methods that can be addressed through qualitative research, and 2) assessing the strengths and limitations of qualitative research in relation to a specific research question.

The focus on assessment may seem too narrow and lacking appreciation for the fact that content, concepts, and skills diffuse throughout an entire course and are therefore difficult to isolate. However, the CEPH model does help instructors (and instructional designers, where available) be intentional about content and evaluation and make sure that course goals are met. No one wants disappointed students who didn't get what they signed up (and paid!) for.

Even if a program is not CEPH-accredited, reviewing an allied accrediting body's competency, content, and evaluation requirements can be a helpful starting place when thinking about how to design evaluations.

Authentic assessment

Authentic assessment asks students to perform tasks that simulate real-world scenarios, and that demonstrate a meaningful application of essential knowledge and skills. When possible, we incorporate authentic assessment into our courses, as it encourages a stronger connection to that knowledge and skill and affirms our commitment to training public health practitioners and researchers who are well versed in translating research to practice and engaging in practice-informed research. However, as we acknowledge later in this chapter, authentic assessment may require more resources— both time and skilled assessors who are knowledgeable about the assessment's didactic underpinnings. Some of this chapter's sample assessments are authentic (e.g., developing and applying a coding scheme, conducting an interview, writing a grant proposal); others are not (multiple-choice questions, responding to a prompt on a discussion forum). Many of our courses include both authentic and other forms of assessment.

Our approach to designing and evaluating authentic assessments varies. For example, students can conduct a mock interview or lead a focus group as part of an authentic assessment. Even within an authentic assessment, there are different perspectives from which to evaluate. In one, you assess your students' use of specific interviewing skills, such as whether they ask open-ended questions and use appropriate probes and rapport-building strategies. In another, you might prompt students to evaluate their own performance with a reflective essay describing their strengths and areas for improvement. For the latter, a student will not be penalized when they conducted a bad interview, so long as they recognize their shortcomings and reflect on, say, their leading or closed-ended questions, missed opportunities for follow-up questions, or their feedback to the interviewee that their responses were wrong!

Either approach can be appropriate and effective depending on the assessment activity's role in the overall course. Authentic assessments allow you to give students credit for completing the exercise or assignment with a focus on the process, or to grade the assignment (for example, using a rubric) to determine whether they met specific learning criteria. Your choice should be informed by your teaching philosophy, available resources, and/or institutional requirements. And while completed credit is probably sufficient motivation for most students to engage with the relevant content, graded activities can push your students beyond their comfort zone or increase the likelihood of more prolonged, active engagement with course material and skill-building.

Finally, for some assessments, your extensive written feedback may be appropriate and necessary. However, we acknowledge that providing such feedback is related to the size of the class and the instructional team's capacity and resources. There are many instances in which the best approach may be to design assessments that demonstrate whether students were engaged with the material.

Capacity of instructional team

A course's assessments will depend on many factors, including the format (online or in-person), the size (small seminar or large lecture), and the composition of the instructional team (individual faculty member or faculty and teaching assistants). Assessment type can also depend on the time available to administer and evaluate work completed. Assessments may also incorporate a peer feedback component—an approach that may be particularly well suited for graduate courses.

Interview guides, practice interviews, and initial drafts of qualitative analysis findings might be particularly conducive to peer feedback. Peer assessment can motivate students toward a more deliberate engagement with course material, with a goal of exchanging ideas with other students in explicitly and intentionally nonhierarchical ways. When incorporating peer feedback into assessment processes, taking time to provide guidance and instruction on how to effectively provide constructive feedback is time well spent. Rubrics that establish domains for expected response content and provide examples of how to communicate strengths and weaknesses of particular components of an assignment can guide peer assessors on how to include clear feedback and will go a long way toward creating an environment where peer assessors are skilled and thoughtful, and their comments are well received by those being assessed. Giving and receiving constructive feedback is an important skill that will serve your students outside the classroom as well. By providing a structure for reacting to and improving each other's work through critical self-assessment and reflection, this approach can also empower students to engage more deeply in relation to their own learning while in their degree programs as well as in their careers. Please note that if you are going to include peer assessment as part of your course, clearly stating this intention in course materials and when explaining assignments is critical to helping students make informed decisions about what they are comfortable sharing given that their writing will be read by their peers.

When we first started teaching large courses (50+ students), we were urged to structure assessments to allow for automated grading (namely, multiple-choice quizzes). We initially balked, thinking that it would be impossible to develop questions that allow us to determine understanding (and not just in terms of retaining terminology). However, we now include structured exams or quizzes in some of our courses regardless of size. Our in-person courses sometimes have closed-book proctored exams; online courses can have remote proctors, although they generally do not, as the arrangement creates considerable practical challenges for students. Instead, for our online offerings, we tend to schedule open-book, time-limited exams and inform students that they won't have time to look up every answer.

By now, we have built a sizeable question bank that we are quite comfortable with, and we value how quizzes grant us real-time insight into ideas and concepts that might need additional attention in the course. Quizzes also free up time for the instructional team to give substantive feedback on written assignments that assess more complex learning objectives. Accounting for an instructor's (or team's) capacity to align with course learning objectives can improve the likelihood that your course's assessments will meet or exceed students' expectations.

Helping students learn

In addition to measuring student mastery, assessments can be powerful learning tools. When used strategically, assessments can promote a deeper understanding and greater retention of material. Formative assessments like quizzes enable students to gauge their comprehension and identify areas of weakness, guiding their studies and engagement with the instructional team. Timely feedback on assessments helps learners recognize and correct mistakes and fosters a growth mindset. Moreover, summative assessments, like final exams or projects, encourage students to consolidate their knowledge and synthesize information—and because the prospect of a comprehensive assessment encourages consistent and sustained learning, they can also motivate learners to engage with the course content throughout.

Assessments can be applied as learning tools to a range of types and modalities—from take-home exams to classroom-based activities. Classroom Assessment Techniques (CAT; Daas &

McBride, 2014) are mechanisms for encouraging students to consider an activity's effect on their knowledge, perceptions, or likely future actions and, in so doing, for assessing the extent to which they understand the material. One example of a CAT is a one-minute paper followed by a Think-Pair-Share exercise to use formative assessment as a strategy for reflecting upon students' understanding of key concepts. Because Think-Pair-Share format encourages active participation, engagement, and peer-to-peer teaching and learning, observing the responses and discussions during the "Share" activity can provide instructors with valuable insight into the students' grasp of the material and let them adjust their teaching accordingly. In addition, this activity promotes critical thinking, communication skills, and the development of metacognitive abilities, all of which contribute to a deeper, more comprehensive understanding of the subject matter and the development of good learning habits.

Types of assessments and examples

It might be tempting to think that because a course teaches qualitative methods, its assessments should also be qualitative. However, as previously indicated, determining the appropriate assessment type means considering many factors. Both qualitative and quantitative assessments are thus fair game for assessment modalities in qualitative courses. Our largest classes have up to 200 students, meaning text-heavy assessments are just not feasible. We've instead developed structured/quantitative assessments designed to assess our students' knowledge of key concepts. Below, we present example assessments and grading rubrics from several of our courses to illustrate the range of possible assessment options.

We've organized this section into **exams and quizzes**, **papers and reflections**, and **skills applications**. Exams and quizzes are most useful to assess whether students know basic concepts and ideas. Papers and reflections can provide insight into the extent to which students understand processes. These assessments can also demonstrate whether students understand how and why decisions about how to conduct qualitative research are made, and whether students can engage with prior work, integrate concepts, and generate new ideas and material. Skills applications, such as designing an interview guide, assess whether students can translate concepts into practice. Where applicable, we provide additional guidance on incorporating these different assessments into in-person and online courses, in courses with different goals and levels, and in courses of varying sizes.

Exams and quizzes

These assessments are aligned with testing students' recall and understanding—the first levels of Bloom's Taxonomy. Because they can cover a broad range of content, multiple-choice quizzes and exams can also assess the breadth of students' knowledge. Given that multiple-choice exams involve minimal writing, you can use them at all levels of learning. Also, the level of skill and time needed to grade these exams means they are a relatively low burden for the instructional team.

When done well, multiple-choice questions can go beyond basic concepts and evaluate all levels of Bloom's Taxonomy (i.e., application, analysis, evaluation, and creation). Writing exams with well-constructed questions and response options that are consistent with established learning objectives is a challenging, time-consuming investment. It is not always easy to come up with incorrect response options that do not confuse students. We learned this when we began offering multiple-choice quizzes and found ourselves being met with reasonable explanations of how students interpreted a response that we intended to be an incorrect option as the correct one. Striking a balance between options that are so obviously incorrect they border on the ridiculous and those that are so nuanced they result in multiple reasonable interpretations takes some trial and error.

Vetted questions have let us establish a question bank into which we make regular deposits and withdrawals as our courses evolve. Box 9.1 includes examples of multiple-choice questions we've used in our courses.

Box 9.1 Tips and tricks: Multiple-choice quiz question examples

---

Course: Qualitative Research Theory and Methods

Format: in-person or online

Typical class size: 60–180

Purpose: provide an opportunity for students to engage with the material and demonstrate their understanding of the course's core concepts

Examples of questions that assess increasingly challenging levels of Bloom's taxonomy

1. You are hired to study stress and job satisfaction among Baltimore City Health Department staff working with mobile syringe exchange services. You decide to spend three months traveling with the mobile van and observing the team's work and interactions. When work is slow, you conduct informal interviews with the team members, letting the conversations unfold naturally, wherever the team member takes them. This type of interview would best be described as:

   A. **unstructured interviews**
   B. semi-structured interviews
   C. observational interviews
   D. structured interviews

2. True or false: An inductive approach to research means you start with a theory and use it to understand your data.

   A. true
   B. **false**

continued

Box 9.1 *continued*

---

3. Read the following abstract. Which of the following methodologies do you think this study most likely followed?

Background: Empathy is an essential attribute of a good doctor. There are multiple dimensions to empathy, yet many medical training curricula focus only on its display. This study aimed to understand medical students' experience learning and developing empathy.

Methods: Six medical students from a single university were interviewed three times each over their final year of medical school. The interviews were largely unstructured and focused on the participants' lived experience with empathy. Bracketing was used to separate the authors' experiences with empathy. Findings came from inductive thematic analysis.

Results: Five major themes characterized empathy in medical training: "The Empathic Process," "Turning Towards Another," "Feeling With Them," "Embodied Living," and "Empathic Consciousness." The students experienced empathy as an emotion, a relationship with another person, and a practical role for a developing physician. They valued authentic patient encounters, focused feedback, and debriefing, which let them process the emotional and physical experiences of empathy.

Conclusions: In addition to teaching communication skills, medical training should focus on students' inner growth. This may be achieved by guiding students through meaningful reflection and open dialogue with supportive mentors.

   A. grounded theory
   B. ethnography
   C. narrative research
   D. case study research
   E. phenomenology

Answers to multiple-choice questions
1. A, 2. B, 3. E

Grading and feedback

When we need to create a quiz or exam, we refer to our question bank and assemble a quiz we can grade quickly, ensuring that students receive timely feedback. Instructors who have teaching assistants can delegate quiz grading, as the act of grading also provides a substantive opportunity to engage with course management. Discussing quiz results in class allows you to revisit material and delve into any concepts that the quiz revealed require additional explanation—and of course, these discussions could involve the teaching assistants if they did the grading. We have come to consider multiple-choice assessments as an important complement to narrative-based assignments.

We have found it useful to pair multiple-choice questions with questions requiring short answer responses. The two formats provide different ways of testing students' proficiency with course material, with short answer questions challenging students to construct responses using their own words. The answers can yield interesting insights into how students relate the material to their own work. See Box 9.2 for additional details about constructing short-answer questions for your exams and quizzes.

Box 9.2 Tips and tricks: Examples of short-answer/open-ended questions within quizzes

Assessment: quiz with both multiple-choice questions and short-answer (3–5 sentence) questions

Course: Qualitative Research Theory and Methods

Format: in-person or online

Typical class size: 60–180

Purpose: provide an opportunity for students to engage with material and demonstrate their understanding of the course's core concepts

continued

Box 9.2 *continued*

Examples

1. You would like to study how people experience symptoms of myocardial infarction (heart attack) and how they decide to seek care. What methodology might you choose to study this topic and why? Justify your choice briefly. [2–3 sentences]

Multiple correct answers are possible, but each should demonstrate the correct application of a qualitative methodology (e.g., grounded theory, ethnography, narrative research, case study research, phenomenology) and apply it to the topic.

2. You are studying social media influencers who share positive portrayals of vaping (e-cigarette use). Compare what information you might get and what questions you might be able to answer if you relied solely on interviews with the social media influencers with information obtained by reviewing and analyzing their social media content—posting, reactions, etc. [4–6 sentences]

The answer should demonstrate the correct understanding of the methods with their specific application to the topic.

Grading and feedback

We want students to be clear and concise in their short-answer responses. Depending on the course level, the questions can be more challenging. (We have found that grading short answers is well within the skill set of advanced doctoral students, should any be on the teaching team.)

We like to combine short-answer and multiple-choice questions in our courses to give students a chance to explain key concepts in their own words. These complementary assessments help with early identification of any students who are struggling with foundational concepts and allow you plenty of time to intervene with additional instruction. If more than a few students miss questions, short answers can also signal the need to review concepts we may have thought we covered sufficiently.

Papers and reflections

Papers and reflective essays are critical components of a qualitative assessment toolkit. To write them, students must be able to think critically, analyze information, and synthesize knowledge. Students cannot be successful without applying their understanding of the subject matter to construct well-reasoned arguments, and to present evidence and draw conclusions from it. Reflective essays can challenge students to assess their own learning and evaluate their experiences, perspectives, and personal development. Hazzan and Nutov (2014) concluded that the value of reflective assignments in qualitative methods pedagogy lies with their ability to build students' capacity for reflexive contemplation—a key qualitative skill.

Similarly, papers and reflective essays can enhance students' writing through clear and coherent articulation of ideas. These assessments can be a venue for students to express their ideas, opinions, and perspectives on a given topic and encourage them to develop their own voice and arguments. Finally, papers and reflective essays are an opportunity for instructors to give constructive feedback through detailed comments and guidance. This feedback loop facilitates student growth and skill development. Box 9.3 includes an example of a memo-writing exercise we use in one of our classes. The assignment provides a tool for assessing students' ability to demonstrate their understanding of the material through critical analysis and provides an opportunity to read published articles. Table 9.1 is the rubric we use to assess students' responses.

Box 9.3 Tips and tricks: Example assessment comparing two qualitative research articles

---

Course: Qualitative Reasoning
Format: in-person or online
Typical class size: 40–100

continued

Box 9.3 *continued*

Purpose: assess published qualitative research by applying the concepts learned in class

Assignment instructions: For this final assignment, please choose a pair of articles from the two sets provided. Each pair addresses the same health topic but uses different qualitative approaches to answering the research questions. Then, referencing the pair you selected, respond to the following five questions. If your articles offer little direct evidence to inform your answer, you may use indirect evidence to support your response. Each answer should be in paragraph form and no longer than 200 words.

1. How does each article use iterative design?
2. How does each article incorporate reflexivity?
3. What sampling strategy does each article use?
4. What approach to analysis does each article use?
5. What aspects of study rigor do you see in each article?

Grading and feedback

We grade student responses based on the quality of their answers; we operationalize "quality" as a complete response to the question that also demonstrates critical thinking as specified in the associated rubric. We tend to use papers and reflective essays to assess our students' ability to apply and integrate content from the entire trajectory of the course. Thus, assigning papers and reflective essays after quizzes amounts to a check: that the students' foundational knowledge is well established. This check has worked well for our courses and results in assessments that progress along Bloom's Taxonomy over the duration of the term. And, as we stated above, we find that advanced doctoral students are well qualified to grade these exams (given guidance and oversight from faculty). A secondary benefit is that these grading assignments add to the teaching assistants' understanding of the material and their skill set. Sharing substantive grading tasks is a value-add for anyone preparing for (or simply considering) a teaching (or research and teaching) career.

Table 9.1 Grading rubric for two-article comparison

Outstanding (100%)	Very good (90%)	Average (80%)	Poor (70%)	Unacceptable (60%)
The answer responds *fully* to the question and is well justified, with evidence from the articles. The answer demonstrates substantial evidence of critical thinking and synthesis.	The answer responds *mostly* to the question and is justified with evidence from the articles. The answer demonstrates moderate evidence of critical thinking and synthesis.	The answer responds *partially* to the question and is somewhat justified with evidence, though the justification is not compelling. The answer demonstrates minimal evidence of critical thinking and synthesis.	The answer responds *partially* to the question and indicates a lack of understanding of basic course concepts.	The answer is incomplete, with little or no justification, and demonstrates a lack of understanding of basic course concepts.

Skill-building and application

Skills applications through which students develop tools or products used in qualitative research (e.g., interview or focus group guides, coding dictionaries, analysis plans) are a form of authentic assessment. Such tasks evaluate practical competencies and require students to demonstrate how they *use* their knowledge, not just that they know it. As these assignments often mirror real-world tasks and challenges, they can prepare students for professional responsibilities—an important consideration, given that we train both researchers and practitioners in our schools of public health. Instead of having students regurgitate information in a format unlikely to be replicated after they complete their degrees, skills-based assessments require students to use what they've learned to solve problems, create a tangible product (e.g., an interview guide, Box 9.4), or make and justify decisions for advancing a research agenda.

These assessments can also encourage student creativity and innovation such that students increase their engagement with course content. Skills-based assessments often require a degree of self-directed learning; students must plan, execute, and manage their projects (which may in turn require more detailed instruction and added progress reports or check-ins for undergraduate courses). The feedback you give your students as they develop their products and on their final assignment can be a valuable guide for them to refine their skills and translate them into viable future products.

Box 9.4 Tips and tricks: Assessment to develop an in-depth interview guide

Course: Introduction to Qualitative Research Methods
Format: in-person
Typical class size: 20–40
Purpose: apply knowledge of the interview as a data collection tool to develop an in-depth interview guide

Assignment instructions

As part of a grant application, you propose to conduct a series of in-depth interviews. The instructions indicate that you should include data collection tools as application appendices. Develop an in-depth interview guide you will use if your grant proposal receives funding. The interview should take about one hour to conduct and reflect the principles and practices of good interviewing that you learned in the course.

Grading and feedback

For this assignment, our detailed feedback includes supportive comments on student guides and indicates when students have done a good job applying principles they learned in class. For example, we would note if and when the student builds in rapport-building questions at the start of the interview, includes probes that follow questions, and develops a set of questions reasonable for the assignment's one-hour interview time frame. In contrast, we would provide constructive criticism when a guide misses an opportunity to practice principles of good in-depth interviewing by asking mostly closed-ended questions, designing a guide without a seemingly logical flow, or including too many or too few questions for the time constraint. The interview guide is a student's chance to show how well they understand the interview's role in qualitative data collection and how they put their understanding into practice.

The following are examples of the types of feedback we've given on in-depth interview guides. Tailoring your feedback to match your course's instruction will likely improve your students' understanding of your comments and their receptivity to making your suggested changes.

Examples of feedback

The guide flows logically and connects well to the study aims for the project. Some of the questions appear to be repetitive (e.g., questions 2 and 4 both address x; questions 6 and 10 both address y). Consider ways to distinguish these questions from one another.

The number of questions appears to match well with the time allotted for the interview. Additional attention to how some of the questions are asked (see suggested edits to questions 2, 5, and 6) and the inclusion of probes (particularly for question 4 and 9—see suggested language for probes) would further strengthen the guide.

Many of your questions invite open-ended responses consistent with best practices for qualitative interviewing. There are a few questions that, with minor modifications, would likely yield richer data; please see the suggested edits on your interview guide for questions 1, 4, and 7. As you will see from my comments, most of the suggestions address your current questions' leading wording. Ensuring that you don't direct

continued

> **Box 9.4** *continued*
>
> *interviewees to a particular response based on how you ask your question is an important skill.*
>
> *I appreciate your detailed development of your interview guide. The number of questions you included, however, will likely require many more hours than you have to conduct the interview. One way to reduce them is by grouping similar questions and replacing them with a single broader question. (See how I demonstrated this technique on page 2 of your interview guide.)*
>
> *Great job with your opening rapport-building questions. You're off to a strong start!*

Discussion forums and asynchronous online tools

The prior examples can be used in any class format (e.g., in-person, synchronous remote, asynchronous remote). There are also tools specific to online and remote learning that you can incorporate into your assessment strategies. Integrating online discussion tools and course management platforms results in multifaceted benefits for student evaluations and assessments. These platforms provide a structured environment for students to engage in meaningful discourse and allow instructors to evaluate student comprehension of course materials and critical thinking skills. Through discussion formats, students can demonstrate their ability to articulate ideas, defend their viewpoints with evidence, and engage in constructive dialogue with peers. You can assess their interactions to gauge individual contributions, levels of understanding, and adherence to discussion norms, thereby informing your assessment of student participation and comprehension. Additionally, these tools facilitate continuous feedback loops, enabling you to provide timely guidance and encouragement that will improve your students' learning experiences throughout the course. Box 9.5 describes an assignment we designed for a remote course that makes use of the Discussion Forum feature of our online course platform. Through this assignment, we create opportunities for students to engage with one another via response posts. Such opportunities can be particularly important for remote courses where students are not learning in the same physical space.

Box 9.5 Tips and tricks: Assignment to discuss different ways of achieving rigor in qualitative data analysis

---

Course: Using Software in Qualitative Research and Analysis

Typical class size: 20–40

Format: asynchronous online

Purpose: demonstrate an understanding of how different researchers define and apply rigor in qualitative research; articulate an argument in favor of a particular approach

Assignment instructions

Cascio et al. (2019) and MacPhail et al. (2016) have outlined two different approaches to rigor in team-based qualitative data analysis. Which approach do you think qualitative researchers should employ? Why? As a bonus, consider Morse's (1997) assertion that inter-rater reliability is a myth. Do you agree or disagree? Why?

Students will respond to two discussion question prompts posted by the instructional team on the Discussion Forum throughout the course. These prompts will draw on Required Readings and Lectures. To receive credit, responses should indicate clear engagement with the content of the assigned readings or lecture material. In general, students should cite or quote specific passages as a starting point for their response. Doing so will help focus responses on something specific. Then, read and respond to one other student's post.

continued

Box 9.5 *continued*

Some suggested formats for posts include the following:

- direct response to the prompt
- analysis of keywords or concepts
- questions you have about the text or other material—e.g., ideas or concepts that are unclear or confusing, or lines of thought that have further implications
- careful reading of a particular text or discussion material combined with a thoughtful exploration of the multiple possible perspectives, interpretations, or implications of that material
- connections between your thoughts on a given assignment and any points raised by others in the readings or in other course materials

What you should not post:

- casual or flippant remarks
- writing that has not been proofread
- remarks that are mean-spirited, aggressive, or disrespectful to others
- remarks that summarize other students' posts, class lectures, or readings without citation or further analysis

Summary

Grading or assessing work is many instructors' least favorite part of teaching. Nonetheless, when teaching qualitative methods in public health, evaluation is essential to ensuring that students—many of whom will be engaging with the method for the first time and may be more familiar with an objectivist paradigm—don't get lost and can retain knowledge gained. We've developed a diverse array of assessment strategies that allow us to monitor our students' progress with course content in a way that is both effective and helps them build practical skills they can use throughout their degree programs and careers. We hope this chapter's examples will encourage you to embrace assessment as an opportunity to test your students' knowledge and application of course content, influence how you adjust course content to meet learning objectives, and help you to work with students as they develop their qualitative research skills.

Epilogue

Thank you for coming along with us on this journey. It's our pleasure to teach qualitative methods to public health audiences, and we hope that sharing our insights and experiences can help make your own teaching more effective and enjoyable. We intend our brief, concluding chapter to provide parting encouragement and look to the future of qualitative research and pedagogy.

First, remember these lessons for teaching qualitative methods in public health:

- **Qualitative methods are no longer fringe approaches.** Qualitative methods and qualitative analysis are both foundational competencies for public health training and practice, as defined by the Council on Education for Public Health (2016) and the Council on Linkages Between Academic and Public Health Practice (2021). You serve a core public health need by training students in these methods.
- **Be prepared for students with a range of backgrounds and goals.** As we've tried to make clear, it is almost always the case that the student body for public health courses will be heterogenous in background and learning goals. You need to be as explicit as possible about your course learning objectives and build your class sessions around learning structures that introduce concepts for novices while also building upon the experiences of more experienced students.
- **A qualitative methods course needs to engage with theoretical concepts.** Your students will want applicable skills. A good qualitative course also needs to provide students

Teaching Qualitative Research in Public Health. Katherine Clegg Smith et al., Oxford University Press.
© Oxford University Press (2026). DOI: 10.1093/9780197662472.003.0010

with a strong sense of *why* qualitative research is conducted the way it is, as well as *how* to do the research.

- **Embracing qualitative methods doesn't mean rejecting quantitative approaches**. Public health problems are complicated. The data needed to understand and address them can be quantitative, qualitative, or both.
- **Not all qualitative courses can—or should—look alike.** It is important and appropriate to design a course that aims to meet students' needs while accounting for the course audience, course length, course format, number of credits, enrollment, and available resources. The way you structure your course will also depend on how related courses are designed and delivered—as well as on your own capacity, experiences, and interests.
- **...and the same is true of qualitative research**. Qualitative research and qualitative teaching are best approached as an art *and* a science. There aren't definitive rules for conducting qualitative research, nor is there a definitive set of rules for teaching it!

Looking to the future

The future of qualitative research in public health is bright. Qualitative methods have been incorporated into CEPH competencies. Increasingly, colleagues and leadership recognize qualitative methods as a fundamental part of the public health methods toolbox. New technologies, including generative AI, are likely to bring significant advances in textual synthesis—but the core work of insights and interpretation by real people(!) will remain.

Teaching of any kind can be challenging; we also find it incredibly rewarding. Remember: Every struggle is an opportunity for growth for both you and your students. We have found that our students are particularly appreciative and engaged when we share our own research experiences, including times when things did not go according to plan. We encourage you to share as much of your authentic researcher self as possible with your students: Education is more effective when students' learning is experiential and prioritizes problem solving, peer collaboration, and discussion. Not only is it unnecessary for you to prove your rock-solid expertise in every class session, but it's educational when your students see you thinking issues through and being open to learning from them and vice versa.

As an educator, it is important to celebrate small victories, stay curious, and remain committed to fostering a learning environment where students feel empowered to explore and express their perspectives. Effective teaching is an iterative process: Reflect upon what works well; be willing to adapt and innovate based on specific learning environments and objectives. It is just as important to learn from what doesn't work as from what goes well. Provide enough attention to areas of struggle for them to result in insights that can inform your teaching and benefit student learning outcomes.

Don't be afraid to own your course, infusing it with your unique perspective and passion. Tailor your teaching to highlight the aspects of qualitative research that you find most compelling and meaningful. Your enthusiasm can be contagious, inspiring students to develop their own love for qualitative research. Above all, remember that teaching requires a complex blend of knowledge, creativity, empathy, and gumption. None of us get it right every time. But we believe that by picking up this book, you're demonstrating your commitment to doing right by your students.

In doing research for this book, we found several texts that provided guidance on teaching qualitative methods. We include a list of these here, in case they might be of use to you:

- Burnette, D. (1998). *Teaching qualitative research: A compendium of model syllabi.* Council on Social Work Education.
- Hurworth, R. E. (2008). *Teaching qualitative research: Cases and issues.* Sense Publishers.

- Janesick, V. J. (2016). *"Stretching" exercises for qualitative researchers* (4th ed.). Sage Publications.
- Swaminathan, R., & Mulvihill, T. M. (2018). *Teaching qualitative research: Strategies for engaging emerging scholars*. The Guilford Press.

Teaching can be more fun with others

Teaching and conducting qualitative research are enriched by collaboration and community. We're lucky to have had multiple opportunities to team-teach and develop new courses and initiatives together; we also work at a school with a robust qualitative research and educational community. We also realize that many qualitative educators reading this book may feel much more isolated. If this is the case for you, we encourage you to seek out peers both within and outside of your institution, join academic networks, and participate in professional organizations dedicated to qualitative research. Engaging with those who share your passion can provide support, spark new ideas, and generally make your journey more enjoyable and fulfilling. Take advantage of opportunities to involve colleagues—including advanced graduate students—to share your classroom. In addition to the benefit for your students, their guest lectures and skills demonstrations will teach you about their work and in turn help you gain insight into your own practices.

We want to hear from you!

Finally, we extend an open invitation to you to share how you use this book in your teaching. We recognize that because our own set of experiences comes primarily from one institution, it is limited, and so we hope to learn from your diverse and varied experiences. What's worked for you? What were your spectacular fails? We have set up an email for this purpose. Please, reach out to TeachingQualResearch@jh.edu[1] and share with us your experiences, challenges, and successes in teaching qualitative research methods. Your feedback will help us refine our approaches and contribute to the broader community of educators committed to advancing qualitative research education.

---

[1] mailto:TeachingQualResearch@jh.edu

References

Alasuutair, P. (1996). Theorizing in qualitative research: A cultural studies perspective. *Qualitative Inquiry*, 2(4), 371–384.

Altheide, D. (2000). Tracking discourse and qualitative document analysis. *Poetics*, 27, 287–299.

Armstrong, D., Gosling, A., Weinman, J., & Marteau, T. (1997). The place of inter-rater reliability in qualitative research: An empirical study. *Sociology*, 31(3), 597–606.

Bacchi, C. (2009). *Analysing policy: What's the problem represented to be?* Pearson Education.

Bandura, A. (1986). *Social foundations of thought and action: A social cognitive theory*. Prentice Hall.

Barraket, J. (2005). Teaching research method using a student-centred approach? Critical reflections on practice. *Journal of University Teaching & Learning Practice*, 2(2), 17–27.

Beard, J. (2022). *Teaching public health writing*. Oxford University Press.

Becker, H. B. (1993). How I learned what a crock was. *Journal of Contemporary Ethnography*, 22, 28–35.

Biruk, C. (2018). *Cooking data: Culture and politics in an African research world*. Duke University Press.

Bloom, B. S. (1956). *Taxonomy of educational objectives handbook: The cognitive domain*. David McKay.

Blumer, H. (2013). Society as symbolic interaction. In A. M. Rose (Ed.), *Human behavior and social processes* (pp. 179–192). Routledge.

Bosk, C. (2003). *Forgive and remember: Managing medical failure*. University of Chicago Press.

Bowen, G. (2009). Document analysis as a qualitative research method. *Qualitative Research Journal*, 9(2), 27–40.

Bowleg, L. (2008). When Black+ lesbian+ woman≠ Black lesbian woman: The methodological challenges of qualitative and quantitative intersectionality research. *Sex Roles*, 59, 312–325.

Bowleg, L. (2017). Towards a critical health equity research stance: Why epistemology and methodology matter more than qualitative methods. *Health Education and Behavior*, 44(5), 677–684.

Braun, V., & Clarke, V. (2006). Using thematic analysis in psychology. *Qualitative Research in Psychology*, 3(2), 77–101.

Braun, V., & Clarke, V. (2021). *Thematic analysis: A practical guide*. Sage.

Burnette, D. (1998). *Teaching qualitative research: A compendium of model syllabi.* Council on Social Work Education.

Cascio, M. A., Lee, E., Vaudrin, N., & Freedman, D. A. (2019). A team-based approach to open coding: Considerations for creating intercoder consensus. *Field Methods, 31*(2), 116–130.

Centers for Disease Control and Prevention. (2023). *Plain language materials and resources.* https://www.cdc.gov/healthliteracy/developmaterials/plainlanguage.html

Charmaz, K. (1999). Stories of suffering: Subjective tales and research narratives. *Qualitative Health Research, 9*(3), 362–382.

Closser, S. (2010). *Chasing polio in Pakistan: Why the world's largest public health initiative may fail.* Vanderbilt University Press.

Coffey, A., & Atkinson, P. (1996). *Making sense of qualitative data: Complementary research strategies.* Sage Publications.

Connell, R. (2013). *Gender and power: Society, the person and sexual politics.* John Wiley & Sons.

Conrad, P. (1992). Medicalization and social control. Annual review of Sociology, 18(1), 209–232.

Crenshaw, K. (1989). *Demarginalizing the intersection of race and sex: A black feminist critique of antidiscrimination doctrine, feminist theory and antiracist politics. University of Chicago Legal Forum,* (1), 139–167.

Creswell, J. (2016). *30 essential skills for the qualitative researcher.* Sage Publications.

Creswell, J., & Poth, C. (2017). *Qualitative inquiry and research design.* Sage Publications.

Crotty, M. (1998). *The foundations of social research: Meaning and perspective in the research process.* Sage Publications.

Daas, K., & McBride, C. (2014). Participant observation: Teaching students the benefit of using a framework. *Communication Teacher, 28*(1), 14–19.

Dalglish, S. L., Khalid, H., & McMahon, S. A. (2021). Document analysis in health policy research: The READ approach. *Health Policy and Planning, 35*(10), 1424–1431.

Daniel, B. K. (2018). Empirical verification of the "TACT" framework for teaching rigour in qualitative research methodology. *Qualitative Research Journal, 18*(3), 262–275.

Delyser, D. (2008). Teaching qualitative research. *Journal of Geography in Higher Education, 32*(2), 233–244.

Emerson, R. M., Fretz, R. I., & Shaw, L. L. (2011). *Writing ethnographic fieldnotes.* University of Chicago Press.

Fadiman, A. (2012). *The spirit catches you and you fall down: A Hmong child, her American doctors, and the collision of two cultures.* Macmillan Press.

Farmer, P., Nizeye, B., Stulac, S., & Keshavjee, S. (2016). Structural violence and clinical medicine. *Understanding and applying medical anthropology,* 336–343.

Fetterman, D. M. (1998). Ethnography: Step-by-step. Sage Publications.

Foucault, M. (1998). *The History of Sexuality Vol. 1: The Will to Knowledge.* Penguin.

Gale, N. K., Heath, G., Cameron, E. Rashid, S., & Redwood, S. (2013). Using the framework method for the analysis of qualitative data in multi-disciplinary health research. *BMC Medical Research Methodology*, 13, 1–8.

Gerth, H. H., Weber, M., & Mills, C. W. (2013). *From Max Weber: Essays in sociology*. Routledge.

Glaser, B. G., & Strauss, A. L. (1965). Awareness of dying. Aldine.

Glaser, B., & Strauss, A. (1967). *The discovery of grounded theory: Strategies for qualitative research*. Sociology Press.

Goffman, A. (2014). *On the run: Fugitive life in an American city*. University of Chicago Press.

Gold, R. L. (1958). Roles in sociological field observations. *Social Forces*, 36(3), 217–223.

Green, J., & Thorogood, N. (2004). *Qualitative methods for health research*. Sage Publications.

Greenhalgh, T., Annandale, E., Ashcroft, R., Barlow, J., Black, N., Bleakley, A., ... & Ziebland, S. (2016). An open letter to The BMJ editors on qualitative research. *BMJ*, 352, i563. https://www.doi.org/10.1136/bmj.i563

Grodal, S., Anteby, M., & Holm, A. L. (2021). Achieving rigor in qualitative analysis: The role of active categorization in theory building. *Academy of Management Review*, 46(3), 591–612.

Guba, E. G., & Lincoln, Y. S. (1994). Competing paradigms in qualitative research. *Handbook of Qualitative Research*, 2(163–194), 105.

Guest, G., Bunce, A., & Johnson, L. (2006). How many interviews are enough?: An experiment with data saturation and variability. *Field Methods*, 18(1), 59–82.

Guillemin M., & Gillam L. (2004). Ethics, reflexivity, and "ethically important moments" in research. *Qualitative Inquiry*, 10(2), 261–280.

Hammersley, M. (2013). What is qualitative research? Bloomsbury Publishing.

Hammersley, M., & Atkinson, P. (2019). *Ethnography: Principles in practice*. Routledge.

Hazzan, O., & Nutov, L. (2014). Teaching and learning qualitative research ≈ conducting qualitative research. *Qualitative Report*, 19(24), 1–29.

Hennink, M. M., Kaiser, B. N., & Weber, M. B. (2019). What influences saturation? Estimating sample sizes in focus group research. *Qualitative Health Research*, 29(10), 1483–1496.

Hurworth, R. E. (2008). *Teaching qualitative research: Cases and issues*. Sense Publishers.

Janesick, V. J. (2016). *"Stretching" exercises for qualitative researchers* (4th ed.). Sage Publications.

Jarvinen, M. (2000). The biographical illusion: Constructing meaning in qualitative interviews, *Qualitative Inquiry*, 6(3), 370–391.

Kawulich, B. (2016). The role of theory in research. In M. Garner, C. Wagner, & B. Kawulich (Eds.), *Teaching research methods in the social sciences* (pp. 37–47). Routledge.

LaDonna, K. A., Artino, Jr., A. R., & Balmer, D. F. (2021). Beyond the guise of saturation: Rigor and qualitative interview data. *Journal of Graduate Medical Education, 13*(5), 607–611.

Lincoln, Y., & Guba, E. (1985). *Naturalistic inquiry.* Sage Publications.

Link, B. G., & Phelan, J. C. (1995). Social conditions as fundamental causes of disease. *Journal of Health and Social Behavior,* (Special Issue), 80–94.

Loder, E., Groves, T., Schroter, S., Merino, J. G., & Weber, W. (2016). Qualitative research and The BMJ. *BMJ, 352,* i641. https://www.doi.org/10.1136/bmj.i641

Lowe, A., Norris, A. C., Farris, A. J., & Babbage, D. R. (2018). Quantifying thematic saturation in qualitative data analysis. *Field Methods, 30*(3), 191–207.

MacPhail, C., Khoza, N., Abler, L., & Ranganathan, M. (2016). Process guidelines for establishing intercoder reliability in qualitative studies. *Qualitative Research, 16*(2), 198–212.

Maietta, R., Mihas, P., Swartout, K., Petruzzelli, J., & Hamilton, A. B. (2021). Sort and sift, think and shift: Let the data be your guide. An applied approach to working with, learning from, and privileging qualitative data. *The Qualitative Report, 26*(6), 2045–2060.

Malterud, K., Siersma, V. D., & Guassora, A. D. (2016). Sample size in qualitative interview studies: Guided by information power. *Qualitative Health Research, 26*(13), 1753–1760.

Marshall, C., & Rossman, G. B. (1989). *Designing qualitative research.* Sage Publications.

Maxwell, J. A. (2005). *Qualitative research design: An interactive approach* (2nd ed.). Sage Publications.

Maykut, P., & Morehouse, R. (1994). *Beginning qualitative research: A philosophical and practical guide.* Routledge.

McTighe, J., & Wiggins, G. (2012). *Understanding by design framework.* Association for Supervision and Curriculum Development.

Miles, M. B., & Huberman, A. M. (1994). *Qualitative data analysis: An expanded sourcebook.* Sage Publications.

Miles, M., Huberman, A., & Saldaña, S. (2019). *Qualitative data analysis: A methods sourcebook* (4th ed.). Sage Publications.

Miller, G. (1997). Contextualizing texts: Studying organizational texts. In G. Miller & R. Dingwall (Eds.), *Context and method in qualitative research* (pp. 77–91). Sage Publications.

Mills, C. W. (1959). *The sociological imagination.* Oxford University Press.

Morgan, D. (1997). *Focus groups as qualitative research* (2nd ed.). Sage Publications.

Morse, J. (1997). "Perfectly healthy, but dead": The myth of inter-rater reliability. *Qualitative Health Research, 7*(4), 445–447.

Morse, J. (2015). Critical analysis of strategies for determining rigor in qualitative inquiry. *Qualitative Health Research, 25*(9), 1212.

National Commission for the Protection of Human Subjects of Biomedical & Behavioral Research. (1978). *The Belmont report: Ethical principles and guidelines for the protection of human subjects of research* (Vol. 2). Department of

Health, Education, and Welfare, National Commission for the Protection of Human Subjects of Biomedical and Behavioral Research.

Othman, M. M., Al-Wattary, N. A., Khudadad, H., Dughmosh, R., Furuya-Kanamori, L., Doi, S. A., & Daher-Nashif, S. (2022). Perspectives of persons with type 2 diabetes toward diabetes self-management: A qualitative study. *Health Education & Behavior*, 49(4), 680–688.

Owczarzak, J., & Smith, K. C. (2022). Implications of the Revised Common Rule for qualitative health research: Opportunities, concerns, and recommendations. *Qualitative Health Research*, 32(2), 385–393.

Patton, M. Q. (2002). *Qualitative research & evaluation methods* (3rd ed.). Sage Publications.

Pelto, P., & Pelto, G. (1978). *Anthropological research: The structure of inquiry.* Cambridge University Press.

Peräkylä, A. (2016). Validity in qualitative research. In D. Silverman (Ed.), *Qualitative research* (pp. 413–428). Sage Publications.

Poteat, T., German, D., & Kerrigan, D. (2013). Managing uncertainty: A grounded theory of stigma in transgender health care encounters. *Social Science and Medicine, 84*, 22–29.

Pratt, M. G. (2009). For the lack of a boilerplate: Tips on writing up (and reviewing) qualitative research. *The Academy of Management Journal*, 52(2), 856–862.

Proctor, E., Silmere, H., Raghavan, R., Hovmand, P., Aarons, G., Bunger, A., Griffey, R., & Hensley, M. (2011). Outcomes for implementation research: Conceptual distinctions, measurement challenges, and research agenda. *Administration and Policy in Mental Health and Mental Health Services Research, 38*, 65–76.

Qureshi, K. (2019). *Chronic illness in a Pakistani labour diaspora.* Carolina Academic Press.

Richardson, L., & St. Pierre, E. A. (2005). Writing: A method of inquiry. In N. K. Denzin & Y. S. Lincoln (Eds.), *The Sage handbook of qualitative research* (3rd ed., pp. 959–978). Sage Publications.

Robertson, J. (2002). Reflexivity redux: A pithy polemic on "positionality." *Anthropological Quarterly, 75*(4), 785–792.

Rosenstock, I. (1974). Historical origins of the health belief model. *Health Education & Behavior, 2*(4), 328–335.

Ryan, G., & Bernard, H. R. (2003). Techniques to identify themes. *Field Methods, 15*(1), 85–109.

Saldaña, J. (2015). *The coding manual for qualitative researchers* (3rd ed.). Sage Publications.

Santiago-Delefosse, M. (2016). Quality of qualitative research in the health sciences. *Social Science and Medicine, 148*, 142–151.

Saunders, B., Sim, J., Kingstone, T., Baker, S., Waterfield, J., Bartlam, B., … & Jinks, C. (2018). Saturation in qualitative research: Exploring its conceptualization and operationalization. *Quality & Quantity, 52*, 1893–1907.

Schensul, J., & LeCompte, M. (2012). *Essential ethnographic methods: A mixed methods approach* (2nd ed.). AltaMira.

Seidman, I. (2006). *Interviewing as qualitative research: A guide for researchers in education and the social sciences.* Teachers College Press.

Shawar, Y. R., & Shiffman, J. (2020). Generating global priority for addressing rheumatic heart disease: A qualitative policy analysis. *Journal of the American Heart Association, 9*(8), e014800.

Silverman, D. (2011). Interpreting qualitative data. Sage Publications.

Silverman, D., & Marvasti, A. (2008). Doing qualitative research: A comprehensive guide. Sage Publications.

Smythe, T., Inglis-Jassiem, G., Conradie, T., Kamalakannan, S., Fernandes, S., Van-Niekerk, S. M., English, J., Webster, Hameed, S., & Louw, Q. A. (2022). Access to health care for people with stroke in South Africa: A qualitative study of community perspectives. *BMC Health Services Research, 22*(1), 464.

Solimeo, S. (2009). *With shaking hands: Aging with Parkinson's disease in America's heartland.* Rutgers University Press.

Spradley, J. P. (2016). *The ethnographic interview.* Waveland Press.

Swaminathan, R., & Mulvihill, T. M. (2018). *Teaching qualitative research: Strategies for engaging emerging scholars.* The Guilford Press.

Taquette, S. R., Borges, L. B., & Souza, M. (2022). Ethical dilemmas in qualitative research: A critical literature review. *International Journal of Qualitative Methods, 21*, 1–15.

Taylor, H. A., Rutkow, L., & Barnett, D. J. (2018). Local preparedness for infectious disease outbreaks: A qualitative exploration of willingness and ability to respond. *Health Security, 16*(5), 311–319.

Thambinathan, V., & Kinsella, E. A. (2021). Decolonizing methodologies in qualitative research: Creating spaces for transformative praxis. *International Journal of Qualitative Methods, 20*.

Timmermans, S., & Tavory, I. (2022). *Data analysis in qualitative research: Theorizing with Abductive Analysis.* University of Chicago Press.

Tuhiwai Smith, L. (2013). *Decolonizing methodologies: Research and indigenous peoples.* Zed Books Ltd.

Venkatesh, S. A. (2008). *Gang leader for a day: A rogue sociologist takes to the streets.* Penguin.

Wagner, C., Kawulich, B., & Garner, M. (2019). A mixed research synthesis of literature on teaching qualitative research methods. *Sage Open, 9*(3), 1–18.

Weller, S., Vickers, B., Bernard, H. R., Blackburn, A. M., Borgatti, S., Gravlee, C., & Johnson, J.C. (2018). Open-ended interview questions and saturation. *PLOS One, 13*(6), e0198606.

Wynters, R., Liddle, S. K., Swann, C., Schweickle, M. J., & Vella, S. A. (2021). Qualitative evaluation of a sports-based mental health literacy program for adolescent males. *Psychology of Sport and Exercise, 56*, 101989.

Ziebland, S., & McPherson, A. (2006). Making sense of qualitative data analysis: An introduction with illustrations from DIPEx (personal experiences of health and illness). *Medical Education, 40*(5), 405–414.

Index

For the benefit of digital users, indexed terms that span two pages (e.g., 52–53) may, on occasion, appear on only one of those pages.

Page numbers followed by *f*, *t*, and *b* indicate figures, tables, and boxes, respectively.